# Praise for *The Art of Hypnotic R*

A basic theme for hypnoanalysis is that the client knows what they need, but needs coaching to find it and correct it. Looking beyond activating events or subsequent sensitizing events leads one to the root cause or initial sensitizing events and hence treatment. The psychosomatic problem-solving is artfully described and adjudicated through Roy Hunter's multiple case examples and Bruce Eimer's PTSD and pain patients. Through the techniques that are described in this text, Hunter and Eimer create and activate the art of hypnosis and couple this with an excellent review of various psychotherapy techniques employed.

Hypnoanalysis is truly more art than science and with the strokes of the pen this solid book teaches us to open a new canvas on which those trained in hypnosis arts can paint.

Joseph F. Zastrow, MD,
FAAFP, ASCH President

If you are a therapist reluctant to use regression then read this book as it will encourage you to confidently return to a powerful and misunderstood technique. If you are an experienced regression therapist wondering whether to read this book, do so as it has the potential to open up your perspectives and teach you plenty more.

Peter Mabbutt, CEO/Director of Studies,
London College of Clinical Hypnosis

Informative, well written and with a systematic approach that shows us that, by following the guidelines in this book, hypnotic regression therapy can be a very powerful tool that can be safely used.

Bruni Brewin, President Emeritus,
Australian Hypnotherapists' Association

All clinicians using hypnosis are encouraged to read this work whether as an aid to manage unanticipated spontaneous regressions or as a ready reference for intentionally planned therapy. One's knowledge of clinical hypnosis is incomplete without the foundation of HRT that the authors impart.

Dr. Gabor Filo, DDS, DABHD, FASCH, FPFA

Two of hypnotherapy's stellar practitioners, Roy Hunter and Bruce Eimer, have pooled their expertise to produce a book on regression hypnotherapy so comprehensive, it is the only guide to regression hypnosis a hypnotherapist will ever need.

Judith E. Pearson, PhD, LPC, Hypnotherapist and NLP Trainer, Motivational Strategies, Inc., Springfield, Virginia

As a hypnoanalyst for many years, I can vouch for the fact that this wonderful book contains every bit of information needed to use regression therapy successfully. Scripts, techniques, "how-to" examples and case studies, along with a defined structure for the therapy, make this the ideal read for the newcomer to regression work, as well as having much of worth to those more experienced. Authors Roy Hunter and Bruce Eimer are experienced and accomplished professional therapists – and it shows.

Terence Watts, MCGI, Fellow of the Royal Society of Medicine

This book, meticulous in writing and obviously close to the authors' hearts, is an outstanding credit to them. They have shared generously their wealth of knowledge and their belief in HRT shines through. Enjoy and learn.

Tom Barber DHp, MA, Director, Contemporary College of Therapeutic Studies, UK Co-author of *Thinking Therapeutically: Hypnotic Skills and Strategies Explored*

I recommend this book to all serious students and practitioners of hypnotic regression therapy, and I wish it had been available earlier on in my career as a hypnosis professional. It is an excellent way to make the leap from working as a script bound, direct suggestion hypnotist, to one of being a powerful change maker who can get results when other lesser forms of hypnotherapy have failed.

Cal Banyan, MA, DNGH,
Creator of 5-PATH® Hypnotherapy and 7th Path Self-Hypnosis®

Age regression is a very complex subject. The authors have made it easy to understand by all practitioners of hypnotherapy regardless of the level of their experience and knowledge.

A. Max Chaumette, Jr, MD, ABA, ABMH

**Note: Full reviews from all these professionals can be viewed on the Crown House website www.crownhouse.co.uk**

# THE ART OF HYPNOTIC REGRESSION THERAPY

# THE ART OF HYPNOTIC REGRESSION THERAPY

## A Clinical Guide

C. Roy Hunter, MS, CHt
Bruce N. Eimer, PhD, ABPP

Crown House Publishing Limited
www.crownhouse.co.uk
www.crownhousepublishing.com

First published by
Crown House Publishing Ltd
Crown Buildings, Bancyfelin, Carmarthen, Wales, SA33 5ND, UK
www.crownhouse.co.uk
and
Crown House Publishing Company LLC
PO Box 2223, Williston, VT 05495, USA
www.crownhousepublishing.com

First printed 2012, reprinted 2017.

British Library Cataloguing-in-Publication Data
A catalogue entry for this book is available from the British Library.

ISBN 978-184590851-5 (print)
ISBN 978-184590852-2 (mobi)
ISBN 978-184590853-9 (ePub)
LCCN 2012937015

Printed and bound by
Gomer Gress, Llandysul, Ceredigion

I dedicate my share of this book in loving memory to my sister, Roberta Hunter Kenney (1939–2011), who believed in seeing the best in people. She was a veteran who met and married her husband, Jerry, while serving in the Marine Corps. Years later, their love of people motivated them to give another two years of their lives serving in the Peace Corps.

*C. Roy Hunter*

I dedicate this book in loving memory to my father, Joe Eimer (May 10, 1913–September 4, 1996). Born in Poland and raised in Vienna, he was a survivor of the Nazi Holocaust. Surviving trauma and loss, he came to America with his brothers seeking a new life, but he never forgot where he came from. An active and energetic man, he built a new life and family in America while remaining connected to what was left of his family of origin, which had been decimated by the Nazis. Despite the traumas of his youth, my father was a warm, loving, sacrificing, and ambitious man who knew how to turn adversity to advantage.

*Bruce N. Eimer*

# Acknowledgements

I, Roy Hunter, wish to first express my deepest gratitude for my late mentor and friend, Charles Tebbetts, who taught me the basics of client centered hypnotherapy and regression therapy. Additionally, as Dr. Eimer stated, it takes many people to bring a book like this into print, so I echo his gratitude and praise for all the people at Crown House Publishing who have worked with both of us. Also, I appreciate my wife, Jo-Anne, for her patience during the many late nights I spent writing and revising my contributions to the book. Last but not least, I wish to thank both the hypnosis professionals and hypnotherapy instructors around the world who believe in my work enough to purchase my other books, as well as my clients over the years whose successful results validate the benefits of the client centered approach to hypnotherapy.

*C. Roy Hunter*

Bringing a book like this to fruition demands the help of many people. First, we gratefully acknowledge the expert help, patient assistance, and continual support of our editors at Crown House, Mark Tracten, Rosalie Williams and Beverley Randell, who made this project possible. We gratefully acknowledge David Bowman of Crown House for seeing the value in this book.

I gratefully acknowledge my two mentors in hypnoanalysis and hypnotic regression work, Dabney Ewin, MD and the late David Cheek, MD. Dr. Ewin has been a good friend and mentor for over 20 years. I also thank my mentor and good friend, Jordan Zarren, LCSW, for his friendship and all of the mentoring in hypnotherapy he has provided me over the years. I thank my wife, Andrea, and my daughters, Marisa and Allison, for loving and standing by me over the years, and my mother Cecile Eimer for being there for me my entire life. Last but not least, I thank all of the patients who have shared their life stories with me over the years.

*Bruce N. Eimer*

# Foreword

Hypnosis is a level of focus that allows the person experiencing it to become almost completely unaware of the multiple other things that might otherwise flit in and out of mind. The person in deep tears over a lost love is experiencing hypnosis, as is the person who has unintentionally clicked off into a daydream state during a boring talk. No Olympic weightlifter would lift a weight in competition without being in a state of hypnosis. The mind of the weightlifter is singly focused on lifting the weight, without thoughts of, "I hope my parking meter has enough change in it," or "On my way back I need to pick up some bread."

Hypnosis is a natural state that we all enter spontaneously, and, in itself other than providing some time of focused retreat, it has no special healing properties. But, in the hands of a professional hypnotherapist that hypnotic state of single minded focus can facilitate more rapid wanted change. Hypnosis can also be used by the well trained therapist to gain access to parts that hold unresolved issues; unresolved issues that sometimes bring forth feelings of fear or rejection. That is what this book is about.

This is a book written by two skilled professionals who share methods to gain access to personality parts that need resolution. Things happen in our past that can continue to affect us in our present. That is the central tenet of psychodynamic psychotherapy. It was Freud's understanding of this basic concept that allowed him to become widely known as the father of psychotherapy. Freud saw in his patients a connection between past traumas and the current feelings of being out of control, and he was correct in this vision. What he lacked was an elegant and streamlined therapeutic mechanism to relieve the trauma of the past so it would no longer interfere in the present. His psychoanalysis was lengthy, relied on interpretations of analysts, and too often proved to be ineffective. Still his work spawned other attempts by psychodynamic therapists such as Jung and Adler to assist patients to gain relief from the traumas of their past. These therapies lacked a way to bring forth the parts of the personality (that held onto trauma) so these personality parts could get the needed assistance to gain relief.

The next big movement in psychotherapy was the humanist phenomenological movement. Person Centered, Gestalt and Existential Therapies were an attempt to assist personality parts to gain healing by being able to be heard and understood. Indeed the word, Gestalt, means whole and it was the purpose of the therapy process to bring out parts that kept the personality from being whole. By encouraging clients to talk about the phenomena that had been difficult or confusing it was assumed that they would gain resolution and then the whole personality could be functional. These therapies lacked both a theoretical understanding of the parts of the personality and regression techniques to assist the therapist to quickly and precisely get to the core of the problem. Too often the wrong part would be the talking part, and only truly gifted therapists could assist clients to speak from the parts that carried fear or rejection and speak to them in a way that brought resolution.

The current major movement in psychotherapy is CBT. The cognitive behavioral movement is a reflection of the symptom-based medical movement. The symptom, not the cause of psychological distress is the focus in this movement. CBT therapists are trained that the past is past and there is no benefit in spending time there. They are trained to work with clients to change the way they think about issues, and to give clients homework so they can practice functioning in a different way. A traumatised part of the personality is not accessed and is not healed. It is left with its trauma while surface parts are taught new ways of thinking and new ways of acting. The proverbial bullet is left in the wound, so complete, cathartic healing cannot be experienced.

These CBT techniques can help clients better deal with life issues and can help clients get through tough times, but they do not facilitate deeper change. The part that feels afraid or rejected continues to hold these feelings. If a fun loving and playful part of the personality experiences an incident where fear or rejection overwhelms this state and if there is no real level of conversation and understanding afterword that state can become Vaded (a state overwhelmed by chronic negative feelings). This Vaded state may come to the surface at any time resulting in the person re-experiencing these same negative feelings of fear or rejection. The techniques presented in this book facilitate the therapist to bring out this Vaded state with regression techniques and help this state heal, thus eliminating the root cause of the negative feelings. The symptoms will automatically change because the previously Vaded state has been assisted to a state of normality. A real benefit of this type of intervention is that this state will again be free to resume its original role of being fun loving and playful. The client will feel more free, and will no longer carry those negative 'out of control' feelings. When a situation arises that would have previously brought out the negative feelings of fear or rejection not only will those feelings not come to the surface, but the client will be able to handle the situation using preferred personal resources.

Another benefit in using the types of techniques presented in this book is that they are very quick. It takes more time to train a client in methods of how to think about and deal with an unwanted symptom than it does to directly go to the cause and resolve it. Some therapists use hypnosis to merely focus on the symptom. Often hypnotherapy is thought of as a way to suggest that things will be different, and because of the power of hypnosis it is often thought that things will be different merely because the suggestion was made. Attempting to use hypnosis it this way is like using a smart phone to hammer in a nail. It might work a little, but not very well and, 'what a waste to use such an amazing tool in such a crude fashion.' Rather than make a suggestion that things will be different, leaving the client disempowered, and leaving the client with a suggestion that has not really changed anything about the cause of the problem, it is much better to use hypnosis to help the client to resolve the cause and be able to carry forward with better access to personal resources.

Knowing, understanding and becoming proficient with good regression techniques is a key element in resolving states that are holding onto negative emotions. It is well worth the effort to take the time to add regression techniques to the tool bag of therapeutic skills. Equal emphasis should be taken to become proficient with the techniques to resolve the angst filled states that regression often brings out. The authors present a number of excellent techniques for that purpose.

Hunter and Eimer offer, in this book, tools of discovery, resolution, and power. Rather than simply suggest that things will be different, they provide a way to discover the original sensitizing events that can continue to interfere with clients' lives, they provide methods to assist in the resolution of these states that have held feelings of fear or rejection, and they offer the power for the resolved persons to use their preferred adult states, without the interference of previously angst filled states.

This book is a major addition to the building body of literature that can assist therapists to assist clients to actually resolve issues rather than merely moderate them. It is filled with techniques and underpinning theory that would be useful in any therapeutic practice, and it is thorough in providing techniques from introduction to the conclusion of the session. It is clear that the authors have prepared this book with a purpose for it to be a helpful tool for therapists to assist clients to experience fundamental change. They have achieved their aim.

Gordon Emmerson

# Table of Contents

# List of Abbreviations

AE      activating event

ASCH      American Society of Clinical Hypnosis

CBT      cognitive-behavioral therapy

EFT      Emotional Freedom Techniques

HRT      hypnotic regression therapy

ISE      initial sensitizing event

NLP      neuro-linguistic programming

OBE      out of body

PLR      past life regression

POP      psychoanalytically oriented psychotherapy

PTSD      post traumatic stress disorder

SIE      symptom intensifying event

SPE      symptom producing event

SSE      subsequent sensitizing event

TI      traumatic incident

# Introduction and Overview

Hypnotic regression therapy (HRT) is one of the most valuable hypnotherapy techniques available today; yet it remains one of the most controversial. This is partly due to both psychotherapists and hypnotherapists jumping in without competent training in hypnosis, as evidenced by numerous cases of false memory syndrome over the years.

Because of both the risk of false memories and the potential consequences of mishandling abreactions, anyone using hypnotic regression without knowing how to help clients who experience emotional discharges (i.e., abreactions) is advised to avoid employing regression therapy until properly trained in client centered regression. Sadly, however, a number of professionals criticize hypnotic regression altogether rather than considering the benefits of competent client centered regression therapy. They often mention mishandled regressions—some of which have resulted in litigation—but the critics often fail to acknowledge the untold thousands of clients empowered to resolve their problems after successful regression sessions.

The purpose of this book is to provide important information and guidelines for any hypnosis professional wishing to employ HRT, including a systematic protocol for assisting the client to consciously and subconsciously discover and release the core causes of his/her symptoms and problems.

We have divided the Introduction and Overview into two sections: an Introduction (written by Roy Hunter) and Overview (written by Bruce Eimer). Most chapters are a collaboration of both authors except where otherwise noted.

## Introduction by C. Roy Hunter

Do you know anyone who is uncomfortable getting on an airplane? Over my years of practicing professional hypnosis, most clients who

1

saw me for the fear of flying experienced the success of overcoming the problem rather than simply learning to fly in spite of their anxieties. In fact, some of them became frequent flyers, logging tens of thousands of miles.

The reason is that instead of simply trying to suggest the problem away, I guide the client back in time during a hypnotic regression in order to discover and release the core cause of the fear of flying. Numerous clients seeing me for other problems over the years have also enjoyed success as a result of hypnotic regression therapy; yet in recent years, a number of hypnosis professionals have hotly debated the topic of regression.

The controversy did not come out of thin air. Hypnotic regression therapy enjoyed high popularity for a number of years during the latter half of the 20th century; but even before the end of the 1990s it became the subject of considerable debate. Genuine concerns are at the heart and core of the controversies. Here is a brief summary of the arguments for and against this technique.

Those who use regression often assert that it is very useful in helping the subconscious discover and release the cause of a problem, and that effective use of HRT often achieves lasting results. Those who oppose the use of hypnotic regression techniques usually state one or more of the following reasons for opposing its use: (1) the risk of false memories and/or (2) the belief that clients do not need to experience abreactions (emotional discharges) while remembering unpleasant experiences from their past. Occasionally a third reason is posted, criticizing hypnotherapists who use regression with almost every client. Note that neither of the authors of this book use regression with most of our clients.

This book will explore the concerns about hypnotic regression therapy summarized above, and respond to those concerns by presenting a very workable five-phase protocol for facilitating client-centered hypnotic regression therapy. This protocol was developed by me over a period of years, as described in earlier editions of my hypnotherapy texts (Hunter 1995, 2000, 2007). It is to be distinguished from Cal Banyan's 5-PATH® Hypnosis and Hypnotherapy System. For information about Banyan's 5-PATH®, go to www.5-PATH.com. First, however, we need to define hypnotic regression.

## What is a Hypnotic Regression?

The authors assume that anyone reading this book already understands hypnosis and the hypnotic process. Both my hypnosis students and my clients alike are presented with the concept that *imagination is the language of the subconscious*. Inside your imagination, you have total power and total freedom to be anywhere you wish and to do anything you choose. In addition, we can use the imagination to move through time as well as space.

During a hypnotic state, moving back in time inside the imagination is called a *regression*. As mentioned above, many hypnosis professionals use regression to guide a client back in time in order to discover the cause of a problem. Sometimes people simply wish to remember details about an event. There are also forensic applications of hypnotic regression techniques (briefly overviewed in Chapter 4). While the subconscious does make a record of everything we experience through the five senses, emotions can alter our perceptions, resulting in inaccurate memories.

Unfortunately, a primary reason for the skepticism regarding regression is that many therapists over the years have formed preconceived opinions regarding the causes of problems before hypnotizing their clients, and then proceeded to use regression to validate those opinions. This is inappropriate leading, and is a major cause of what we call "false memory syndrome," which means that a client may believe false perceptions to be facts.

Now let us look at the other side of the coin.

## Hypnotic Regression Therapy Teachers

A number of well-known hypnotherapists have successfully employed hypnotic regression techniques in their clinical practices over a period of many years, with some of their work documented here. My co-author, Bruce Eimer, Ph.D.—a student of Dabney Ewin, M.D. and David Cheek, M.D.—is a licensed clinical psychologist and published author who has used hypnotic regression therapy with numerous clients over the years.

David Cheek, an obstetrician-gynecologist, was a pioneer in the use of hypnotic regression therapy for psychosomatic problems, especially persistent pain syndromes such as chronic pelvic pain and interstitial cystitis, as well as gynecological problems such as infertility. A past president of the American Society of Clinical Hypnosis, Dr. Cheek published a multitude of clinical case reports and literature reviews in the scientific journals, as well as several books on ideomotor signaling and other ideodynamic techniques for facilitating hypnotic regressions and communicating with the patient's unconscious (Cheek, 1993; Cheek & LeCron, 1968; Rossi & Cheek, 1994).

Dabney Ewin, a general surgeon and occupational medicine physician, who was a student of Dr. Cheek, has treated thousands of patients in his over 40 years of hypnosis practice using ideomotor signaling and other hypnotic regression methods. Also a past president of the American Society of Clinical Hypnosis, Dr. Ewin is a pioneer in the use of hypnosis for the treatment of patients with severe acute burn injuries. He has also published many case reports and literature reviews on hypnosis for burns and hypnotic regression therapy for pain, asthma, hives and warts. He also wrote several books on his work (Ewin, 2009; Ewin & Eimer, 2006).

Gil Boyne practiced and taught hypnotic regression therapy for many years and included some case histories in *Transforming Therapy: A New Approach to Hypnotherapy* (1989). I personally witnessed Boyne employing regression therapy to help a stutterer back in the 1980s. A year later, I bumped into that same former stutterer at a hypnosis conference and shared a meal with him. His speech was so clear that one would have difficulty believing that he spent so many years of his life stuttering.

Randal Churchill, a former student of Boyne, chose to specialize in hypnotic regression therapy, and has written two books on this topic. The first one was *Regression Hypnotherapy: Transcripts of Transformation* (2002). He followed with Volume II six years later (Churchill, 2008), and has facilitated many thousands of hypnotic regressions during his career.

Charles Tebbetts, my former mentor, taught hypnotic regression therapy as well, including it in his *Miracles on Demand* (1985). Although he told me personally that he learned regression from Gil Boyne, Tebbetts used a more gentle style that I believe is more client centered.

Dave Elman occasionally used regression, and conducted an astounding session in front of a number of doctors. He claimed, as did David Cheek (1993), that a person in hypnosis could remember something that happened even while totally unconscious—even under anesthesia. Elman hypnotized a physician who had undergone surgery and regressed him back to the operating table where he remembered a conversation taking place during the procedure. As it turned out, his surgeon was one of the doctors present to witness this amazing regression, verifying that the conversation took place (Elman, 1984).

Gerald Kein, known for promoting the work of the late Dave Elman, also teaches hypnotic regression therapy. He taught it to Cal Banyan, a well-known hypnosis instructor, who incorporates regression in his 5-PATH® hypnotherapy program. Banyan has written articles on teaching hypnotic regression (Banyan, 2009) as well as including it in his first book (Banyan & Kein, 2001).

E. Arthur Winkler, Th.D., Ph.D., a Methodist minister with a degree in clinical psychology, conducted exhaustive research on past life regression. He also facilitated thousands of sessions with traditional HRT to a past time in the client's current life to discover and release the cause of the client's problem. To his thousands of students, he emphasized the importance of not practicing beyond their level of training, and the importance of properly guiding, but not leading, their clients.

During Dr. Winkler's lifetime, he hypnotized over 35,000 individual clients and thousands of others in groups. He authored 18 books on the healing power of the inner mind.

Winkler often spoke about Phineas Parkhurst Quimby, who was a 19th century New England clockmaker, inventor and freethinker. In the 1850s, he investigated the "magic" of mesmerism with a skeptical eye. Gifted as a clairvoyant, Quimby would sit and teach each patient about the root cause, or triggering cause, of his/her particular disease or problem. He then explained that, because the patient now understood *how* the disease started, they would now be able to get well—and many did get well. His reputation as a healer quickly spread. During a nine year period (1857–1866), Quimby helped 12,000 people become healed from all kinds of diseases of that day. Perhaps even more importantly, he steered 19th century American hypnosis away from mesmerism and toward the mind–body–spirit connection, which is a key to effective regression therapy today. Anyone wishing to research his work may read *Phineas Parkhurst Quimby: The Complete Writings* (1988) or *The Quimby Manuscripts* (1961). Quimby, often referred to as the Father of Modern Thought, could easily be called the pioneer of regression therapy.

Other practitioners over the decades have practiced and taught hypnotic regression in various forms; but this first chapter is not meant to be an in-depth historical discussion, so let us continue. My approach differs somewhat from most others, as explained below.

## Client Centered Hypnotic Regression Therapy

The type of hypnotic regression therapy that I teach is client centered. One entire chapter of my book, *The Art of Hypnotherapy* (Hunter, 2010b; originally published in 1994), is devoted to regression therapy, with numerous references to regression mentioned elsewhere in the text. Besides teaching HRT since 1987, I have written numerous articles over the years. My approach is based on the concept that the answers to a client's problem can be found within the inner mind of the client:

Here is my explanation of the difference between client centered hypnosis and therapist-directed trance work. During client centered hypnosis, the client comes up with the answers, provided the hypnotist skillfully uses the art of hypnosis to obtain those answers. This requires width and depth of training in the art of hypnosis.

Therapist-directed hypnosis is far more common around the world, and requires less hypnosis training, because the hypnotist determines whatever he/she thinks is the best solution for the client. Often the hypnotist simply uses a script book after just a few days of training, choosing a script to fit the client's concern. Generic scripts help some of the people some of the time, but often leave much undone. (Hunter, 2005: 24)

This is true, regardless of whether the facilitator employs regression therapy or parts therapy. My approach to HRT is organized into five phases:

Phase 1: Client preparation
Phase 2: Regression techniques to discover the cause
Phase 3: Abreactions and release
Phase 4: Subconscious relearning (or reprogramming)
Phase 5: Concluding the session

This phase-by-phase protocol or process makes it both easier to learn hypnotic regression therapy, and easier to teach it. Later chapters of this book explore each phase of HRT in depth, along with some effective techniques along the way. The early chapters discuss some important background information, the difference between leading and guiding, anxieties about false memories and other concerns.

One important objective of this book is to provide the hypnosis professional with a working foundation and discipline for effective use of client centered HRT through each phase of the process. The hypnosis professional experienced with hypnotic regression therapy might know several effective techniques that may appear to be overlooked in these pages; but the goal is not to discuss every possible technique employed. Rather, it is to provide the hypnosis professional with enough information to enable the reader to do his/her own research, and to use the information in a way that works.

The sample scripts provided are like training wheels, designed to serve you, the clinician, and not vice versa. If you find another effective way of obtaining results, go for it. There is more than one way to go from Los Angeles to New York. The destination is more important than the specific details of the journey.

What the following chapters present may not be the only effective way of facilitating client centered hypnotic regression therapy; but experience demonstrates the value of this discipline with clients. The next chapter will examine what I consider to be the foundation of successful client centered hypnotherapy: *the four hypnotherapeutic steps to facilitate change.* I also call these *the four hypnotherapy objectives* or the *four cornerstones of successful hypnotherapy* Accomplishing all four hypnotherapy objectives will increase the probability of lasting success for clients (Hunter, 2005, 2010b). If you already have one of the previous two books mentioned, you may skip Chapter 1, or simply use it for reference; but first, please read the Overview below.

## Overview by Bruce Eimer

I have been using hypnosis as a tool in my psychotherapy practice for over 25 years. Early on, my uses of hypnosis were confined to formal induction and direct suggestion. At first, I relied on scripts and rapidly realized that "scripto-therapy" was quite limited. Therefore, I would read scripts several times and then deliver them in my own words to the client. This allowed me to concentrate on the client and watch their responses closely. This is where a therapist's attention should be—on the client and not on a piece of paper; that is, client centered.

As I developed clinical experience working with clients and using hypnosis, I began to see the limitations of direct suggestions. I took training in Ericksonian and neo-Ericksonian, indirect and conversational hypnosis methods along with Bandler and Grinder's neuro-linguistic programming (NLP), and I began to incorporate these techniques in my work. As a result, I found that my rapport with clients improved, and so did my results. However, because I am always searching for newer and better methods of helping clients get well, I was not satisfied.

In my graduate schooling, I was trained in the cognitive-behavioral therapies, called CBT (Beck 1979; Ellis & Harper, 1975; Lazarus, 1989), as well as psychoanalytically oriented psychotherapy (POP). Both approaches to psychotherapy emphasize the importance of uncovering the client's underlying core and blocking beliefs that give rise to their anxieties and symptoms. Unfortunately, POP is usually a long process that requires years to form a working relationship with the patent, analyze the transferences that develop in that relationship and relate it to the client's neurotic symptoms and core relational problems. Nowadays, we seldom have the luxury of this amount of time to help clients get well. CBT was developed by its innovators in order to make therapy more efficient and less drawn out.

As originally intended, there was the assumption in CBT that by identifying and disputing the client's automatic thoughts and underlying beliefs and adding selective reinforcement based on behavioral principles, dysfunctional emotions and behaviors could be changed. However, the fathers of the first generation of CBT therapies were wise clinicians and they soon realized that something deeper was required. There is an old adage in psychodynamic psychiatry and clinical psychology that it is on Axis II, the personality disorder spectrum of the *Diagnostic and Statistical Manual of Mental Disorders*, that Axis I, the presenting clinical psychiatric disorders such as depression and anxiety disorders, "live." What this means in plain English is that we do not treat disorders. We treat the whole person; the client's personality, both strengths and weaknesses, healthy resources and pathology, influence the onset and the course of the client's emotional and behavioral disorder and symptoms.

Following this realization, the founding fathers of CBT began to move closer and closer to psychodynamic techniques in order to remedy the situation. Things had seemed to come full circle. However, CBT's first practitioners, as well as the upcoming second generation of CBT innovators, still saw limitations in their toolkit. CBT is based upon an active-directive therapist and an active and directed client, as opposed to the more passive and non-directive postures of the more traditionally psychoanalytically trained therapist and client. Therefore, CBT-ers began incorporating hypnosis-like techniques such as guided imagery and relaxation techniques into their practice. The problem was that CBT started becoming much more like script based, direct suggestion hypnosis. All of this I witnessed firsthand as a student of CBT as it developed.

As a result, in my practice, I began to experiment with integrating CBT and direct suggestion hypnosis in order to uncover the client's core automatic thoughts and blocking beliefs in the waking state and then find alternative functional replacement thoughts and beliefs. Then, these positive beliefs were "installed" through suggestion in hypnosis; that is, fixed in place in the client's unconscious. In fact, this is one of the ways I believe that Francine Shapiro developed her brand of waking hypnosis back in 1990; that is, eye movement desensitization and reprocessing (EMDR) (Shapiro, 2011).

The problem I encountered, however, was the same one Sigmund Freud encountered in the 1890s, which led him to drop hypnosis as a tool, and that problem was client resistance. Now, *resistance* is a misleading term. This is because it is real. It exists, but not for the reasons that are on the surface. Most clients do not "not" want to get better. It is just that they are afraid of change and the unknown. Recognize that two negatives (not not) make for a positive. Therefore, the working assumption is that most clients want to get well; but they are afraid of the unknown, and that is why they need a good therapist to help them work through their resistance to being put in a position wherein they might be unable to cope with change. This is an art.

The problem is compounded in my opinion when the therapist thinks he/she knows what is right for the client. This can happen when well-intentioned therapists employing scripted techniques, such as certain forms of CBT and traditional direction suggestion hypnosis, give the client "the answers" or "guide" the client to "the answers." In the case of CBT, this would be in the form of scripted ways to identify and "dispute" dysfunctional thoughts and beliefs, and in the case of hypnosis, this would be in the form of suggestion and imagery scripts. Even Ericksonian and neo-Ericksonian hypnotherapists assume that they know what is best for the client through their use of metaphor and embedded suggestions.

Having gotten to know my co-author, Roy Hunter, and his form of hypnotherapy, I am comforted in knowing that he does not practice this way. He does not presume to know what is best for the client. This is what I believe Roy means when he uses the term "client centered." That is, the answers need to arise from within the client—from the client's inner mind.

Before I met Roy Hunter, my search for better hypnotherapy methods led me to the work of David Cheek, M.D., an obstetrician-gynecologist, a professional hypnotherapist, a hypnosis pioneer and a contemporary and peer of Milton Erickson. Dr. Cheek was a generous and caring human being with a giant intellect. He inspired his students and gave freely of his time. He encouraged me to write my first book, *Pain Management Psychotherapy: A Practical Guide* (Eimer & Freeman, 1996) and to own my own work and confidence. He actually read the early drafts of the manuscript and gave me constructive feedback. I studied with Dr. Cheek for several years by telephone and we corresponded via old-fashioned mail from 1994 through 1996. When I was preparing for back surgery in 1996, he conducted ideomotor hypnoanalysis sessions with me over the telephone and helped me cope with my fears and anxieties to prepare for surgery. The outcome was successful.

Dr. Cheek was a courageous pioneer in the use of hypnotic regression therapy. He was unafraid to embrace the exploration of new and unpopular ideas, and to investigate their validity and utility. Although he was a non-traditionalist, and not a follower, Dr. Cheek was well trained in the traditional medical sciences and in the scientific method. He collaborated with psychologist, professional hypnotherapist and author

Leslie LeCron on the book, *Clinical Hypnotherapy* (1968), and traveled extensively with LeCron conducting hypnosis workshops around the country for physicians and dentists. Cheek and LeCron developed the model of the seven psychodynamic causes or "keys" to psychosomatic symptoms, and the use of ideomotor questioning to explore them, which are mentioned in Chapter 4.

I was personally introduced to the work of Dr. Cheek by Dabney Ewin, M.D. in 1991 at an annual conference in Philadelphia of the American Society of Clinical Hypnosis (ASCH). Dr. Ewin is a surgeon, occupational medicine and emergency room physician in New Orleans. As was Dr. Cheek, Dr. Ewin is a past president of ASCH, and he is also a student of Dr. Cheek. Dr. Ewin has been a pioneer in the use of hypnosis in the emergency room, in the treatment of burns and in the management of pain and other psychosomatic symptoms. Dr. Ewin developed his own brilliant style of doing hypnotic regression therapy and is one of the grand masters in the field of clinical hypnosis. Through Dr. Ewin's generosity, we struck up a personal friendship and I have studied with him for the past 20 years. I helped Dr. Ewin write a book describing his methods called *Ideomotor Signals for Rapid Hypnoanalysis* (Ewin & Eimer, 2006).

I have used the techniques of Dr. Cheek and Dr. Ewin for almost 20 years in my psychotherapy and hypnosis practice. I have found that the "art," as Roy would say, of doing this work lies in how the hypnotherapist uses the material uncovered and brought out through the age regression and ideomotor signaling work. The challenge is something akin to that discussed in good basic hypnosis courses, which raises the question: Now that I have the client in hypnosis trance, what do I do next? There certainly is an art to getting clients there, but the greater challenge is figuring out how to use the material that comes up. The answer comes from a healthy combination of clinical experience, common sense and empathy with the client. In fact, doing HRT helps clinicians to develop empathy with the client as you get to see the world that the client lived in and lives in from the client's point of view. That makes all the difference in the world because typically nobody else can feel your pain. Doing HRT gives you a lens into that

world, and empathy is an essential ingredient for competent and efficient psychotherapy.

Roy's work provides a nuts-and-bolts, phase-by-phase protocol for
working with and helping the client work through the material that
comes up in the hypnotic exploration of their inner world. You cannot use a script to do it. However, you cannot fly by the seat of your
pants or shoot from the hip. As with Dr. Ewin's and Dr. Cheek's protocols, ideomotor questioning, as well as speaking with the client during
the hypnotic age regression session, gives you, the therapist, tips as
to what to ask next and what to say. However, you cannot go into the
session with preconceived notions or assumptions about what is going
to come up. Be prepared to be surprised. That is part of the wondrous
excitement of doing this work.

Hypnotic regression therapy, as we present it here, which is how Roy
has taught it in so many workshops for professional hypnotherapists,
is not scripto-therapy or scripto-hypnosis. Unfortunately, too much
of the controlled psychotherapy and hypnosis research nowadays that
aims at constructing and validating evidence-based therapies is centered on the application of manual-guided and heavily scripted fixed
protocols with carefully selected clients. This limits the external gen-
eralizability and validity of this psychotherapy research. In the real
world, most of us take clients as they present themselves, which is
how they walk into our offices. We do not have the luxury of rejecting
unsuitable candidates. In addition, we endeavor to fit the therapy to
the client rather than the other way around. There are no Procrustean
beds in our offices—thank goodness!

As I have written previously (Zarren & Eimer, 2002), rigid and compul-
sive therapeutic rituals often reinforce dysfunctional behavior if they
are not developed from an adequate case conceptualization. Good case
formulation or conceptualization is "client centered," as Roy puts it.
The good hypnotherapist helps the client to bring up the material that
is lying dormant in the patient's unconscious, although not really dormant because it is not fully processed or digested and thus is blocking
the client from moving on with his/her life in a healthier way.

## "Art" vs. "Science"

Contrary to what the ivory tower establishment purveyors of manualized evidence-based treatment protocols would have you believe, and would make "clinical law," hypnotherapy and psychotherapy entail more *art* than *science*. The art of hypnosis and hypnotherapy, as Roy has discussed in his previous books (Hunter, 2010a, 2010b), entail employing the science of hypnosis and therapy in an individualized manner for each client—weaving together the threads of different techniques and interventions as part of a coherent overall treatment plan. Knowledge about designing a treatment plan is one thing, and it is derived from reading, training, workshops and clinical experience. However, the implementation of the treatment plan is colored by the personality and experiences of the therapist in interactions with the personality, presenting complaints and hidden agenda of the client.

Art is created; and no two works of art are the same. This is also the case with clinical hypnotherapy cases. Each client is different. While clients present with similarities and patterns, individual differences account for much of the variance in terms of who gets better and who does not. The art of hypnotherapy is the art of co-creating different masterful pieces of work in collaboration with each of your unique clients as you consciously employ yourself in the process. To make this happen, you, the therapist, need to formulate a clear case conceptualization that guides your employment and implementation of different hypnotherapy techniques artfully and consciously. This involves the *what do you do* and *what do you say and ask* when you conduct your initial evaluation of the client, when you explain hypnosis, when you induce hypnosis and when you utilize the hypnosis trance to do therapy—hypnotherapy.

Neither Roy nor I advocate practicing with a "cookie cutter" approach. Cookie cutter approaches only work some of the time, and when they do, only with highly motivated clients who present with simple problems. As all experienced clinicians know, the clients we most commonly see in our offices are complex and have conflicting motivations. As Freud said, they have resistance to getting well that must be analyzed. This resistance is their defense mechanisms at work inter-acting with their personality, their life history and their current life circumstances.

## Regression

Milton Erickson (Erickson, Hershman & Secter, 1961) and David Cheek both believed that people "enter hypnosis as they mentally review sequential events." Cheek wrote, "A hypnoidal state is entered when [remembering sequential events such as] recalling a tune, remember-ing the visual images of waves breaking on a beach, the movements of a candle flame, and the words of a poem" (Rossi & Cheek, 1994: 1). Thus, a basic mechanism for inducing a *hypnotic altered state* is the review or processing of a sequence of sensory impressions or mem-ories (Zarren & Eimer, 2002). Of course, the cornerstone of Freud's psychoanalytic approach is the reconstruction, analysis and interpre-tation of the client's childhood. That is hypnotic.

When we remember events, we go back in our minds and, to some degree, re-experience aspects of those events. The degree and inten-sity of our re-experiencing, or *revivification*, is influenced by the degree of emotion associated with the memories. Thus, all therapy to some extent entails the processes of hypnosis, trance and regression, whether or not the therapist formally employs them. Therefore, good therapy and good hypnotherapy should entail the conscious and skill-ful use of regression techniques by the therapist. So, let's now move on to the good stuff.

# CHAPTER 1

# Important Background Information

During the 19th century, our hypnotic pioneers primarily used *prestige suggestion* to obtain results (Quimby, mentioned in the Introduction, was an exception). As the 20th century approached, it became apparent that suggestion alone was usually insufficient to provide permanent benefit to many of the clients of that time; however, the scientific approaches of the era fitted the client to the technique rather than vice versa.

One of the reasons Freud discarded hypnosis was because he grew tired of the monotonous sleep suggestions (Zanuso, 1986). Additionally, he did not believe that deep hypnotic states were necessary in order to achieve results. This might have been a rationalization as Freud had difficulty inducing deep hypnosis in his clients. Perhaps if he had mastered the art of hypnosis, or learned to fit the technique to the client instead of fitting the client to the technique, we would have a very different history of both hypnosis and psychology ... but let us deal with the status of hypnosis today.

First, a hypnotherapist must master basic hypnotic techniques. An outstanding therapist could easily miss an opportunity to help someone make an empowering life change if the client is an analytical resister emerging from trance too soon.

Second, we now have a foundation for hypnotherapists to build a multimodal approach for their clients that incorporates four essential hypnotherapy objectives, discussed later in this chapter.

Third, a professional hypnotherapist should understand how to competently facilitate regression therapy, because some clients spontaneously enter regression when talking about a problem. The important difference between leading and guiding is too important to omit, so an entire chapter is devoted to that topic (see Chapter 2).

Additionally, there are a few other hypnotic techniques, such as ideo-motor signaling and responding, that may often be quite useful in hypnotic regression therapy, which are presented in depth in other books (Cheek, 1993; Ewin & Eimer, 2006; Hunter, 2005). These techniques are mentioned where applicable in this book.

Let us begin with the four essential, or primary, hypnotherapy objectives, which Roy also calls *the four cornerstones of successful hypnotherapy*. He has discussed them in two of his hypnosis texts (Hunter, 2005, 2010b).

## The Four Primary Hypnotherapy Objectives

Certainly hypnotic suggestion and imagery have proven their ability to help *some* of the people *some* of the time, but the authors believe that a competent hypnotherapist can help *most* of the people *most* of the time. We can accomplish this by building our therapeutic approach on a foundation of four primary hypnotherapy objectives:

1. Suggestion and imagery
2. Discover the cause
3. Release (emotional attachment to the cause)
4. Subconscious relearning

We consider these four therapeutic objectives to be the cornerstones of client centered hypnotherapy (see Figure 1), whether accomplished within one hypnotherapy session or across several sessions, especially where subconscious blocking beliefs bound by strong emotions are present. *Effective results often require fulfilling all four objectives.* Both of Hunter's books which mention these cornerstones label them as "the four hypnotherapeutic steps to facilitate change" because Charles Tebbetts (1985) originally used that term.

Now we will discuss each objective individually.

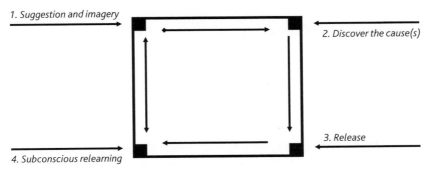

Figure 1. The four primary objectives of hypnotherapy

## Suggestion and Imagery

Every behavior, thought and habit is motivated (i.e., moved, energized or activated) by something. As Freud pointed out in his theory of multiple determinants, there is usually more than one motivator; and often, these motivational determinants are conflicting. Emotion is the experience of these motivators or activators, and is the motivating power (or motion activating energy) of the inner mind.

With a strong motivating desire to change, direct suggestions, imagery and post-hypnotic suggestions (direct or indirect) may be sufficient to provide lasting benefit to some of the clients some of the time (Tebbetts, 1985). Marketers of hotel hypnosis seminars take advantage of this fact and gather enough testimonials to attract thousands more to their traveling seminars. Without a strong desire to change, however, either subconscious or conscious beliefs may block suggestions for positive change. An investigative journalist told one of the authors that he discovered that, on average, only 20% of hotel hypnosis seminar attendees for smokers were able to go more than one week without backsliding into the smoking habit. The problem is that most clients have conflicting motivations about making changes. Therefore, most people need more than just direct suggestion and imagery to create lasting success.

How many people do you know who have been to a hypnotist to stop smoking, only to start up again, often just hours or days after their session? Many smokers backslide even after two or three sessions. This fact validates the theory that all hypnosis is really self-hypnosis. It also demonstrates that the real power to change (or not change) *lies within the client.*

When subconscious resistance exists (and these blockages to change pop up frequently), Objectives 2, 3 and 4 must *all* be addressed and used. The first objective then also becomes the last one—the installation of change facilitating and reinforcing suggestions and images. This is why Roy Hunter considers these objectives to be the *four cornerstones* of successful hypnotherapy. They form the foundation for building long lasting success for your clients (Hunter, 2005).

Even when we know that all four objectives are necessary, it is still advisable to start with the first one. By using suggestions to increase the motivating desire to change, the client is more likely to show up for any necessary subsequent sessions. Additionally, positive suggestion and imagery will usually leave a good impression of hypnosis, and first impressions are lasting.

### Discover the Cause
Note the word "discover" rather than diagnose. First, a hypnotherapist does not diagnose unless licensed to do so. Second, when facilitating client centered hypnosis, the client centered approach is based on the concept that the client's inner mind can reveal the core cause of a problem when we employ appropriate hypnotic techniques. Third, "diagnosis" is often a process of labeling, not analyzing and understanding client centered psychodynamics.

If subconscious resistance exists, there is a reason. We may choose from among a variety of techniques that enable the subconscious to reveal the cause of a problem. Numerous books discuss various techniques for discovering the cause(s) of a client's problem, including (but not limited to) ideomotor responding, hypnotic regression therapy, parts therapy, ego state therapy, voice dialogue, verbalizing and other techniques.

The hypnotherapist employing client centered hypnosis does *not* attempt to determine the cause himself or herself; instead, the therapist asks the client's subconscious for permission to reveal the cause(s). If a therapist reaches a prior conclusion regarding the cause of a client's problem, and then employs direct suggestion hypnosis or other hypnotic techniques such as regression therapy to validate that conclusion, there is a risk of subconscious confabulation and/or false memories. This would be *inappropriate leading*.

For example, if we employ hypnotic regression to "prove" that a client was abused, false memories may easily occur. Whether the therapist forms an opinion about the cause from analytical logic, professional conclusions, intuition, so-called "psychic gifts" and/or religious beliefs, what happens to the client if that opinion is incorrect?

Gordon Emmerson, author of *Ego State Therapy*, states that if *either* the therapist *or* the client has a preconceived opinion regarding the cause of a problem, that opinion would be incorrect 50% of the time (Emmerson, 2003). Are you willing to gamble on those odds? In addition, Randal Churchill warns the clinician about the risk of producing false memories when the therapist operates from a position of certitude about the cause of a client's problem (Churchill, 2002).

Preconceived opinions implanted by the therapist can taint the trance and take the client down the wrong path. Even if the conclusion is a correct one, some other important cause might never emerge during the session. Unfortunately, such inappropriate leading happens in the offices of many mental health counselors and licensed health professionals who use hypnosis, and in some offices of hypnotherapists whose training in regression and hypnotherapy is inadequate. This can result in false memory syndrome, creating emotional hurt as well as legal consequences for family members and/or the therapist (Loftus & Ketcham, 1996). The client centered approach is to find a way to get the client's own mind to disclose the cause.

Once we discover the cause(s) of a client's concern, we must complete the next objective in order to reduce the risk of the client "buying back" the problem.

## Release

Awareness of the cause is not enough for everyone. Many clients will not be able to spontaneously release their bound up emotions which connect them to the problem at a subconscious level, unless asked to do so while experiencing deep hypnosis. During the hypnotic state, the relationship of the cause and its bound up influence to the symptom is more easily established emotionally as well as intellectually. We may then use one or more hypnotherapy techniques to facilitate release.

This often involves forgiveness of self and/or releasing others. Note that we must accomplish the release at a subconscious level and not simply at the conscious level alone. Forgiving does not mean condoning. The words "let it go" or "release it" are often more comfortable than "forgive." Thus, regardless of the wording, it is usually very important that clients also *forgive themselves*; that is, let themselves off the hook that has been crippling them emotionally and/or physically. These words are in fact consistent with the etymology or origins of the term "to forgive." To forgive means "to give up for." We are referring to giving up the emotional attachment to the perceived cause(s) of the current problem for the sake of what is most important to the client— what he holds most dear, including (hopefully!) himself or herself.

Even if not disclosed to the therapist, the subconscious still must discover and identify the cause of the problem in order to release it and have lasting results. In rare instances, the client's conscious mind might not be aware of the cause discovered by the subconscious with very effective indirect suggestions and metaphors; but finger responses can indicate when the inner mind discovers and releases the cause.

Numerous techniques can be used to facilitate release, including (but not limited to) hypnotic regression therapy, Emotional Freedom Techniques (EFT), NLP and hypnotic parts therapy or its variations. However, some NLP and EFT practitioners attempt to release a problem while the cause remains buried in the subconscious, unrecognized and hence unresolved. Note that if the problem is released through any of the above techniques *without* the cause being discovered, understood on an appropriate level and released, the subconscious is fully capable of returning the same problem or another one that is worse (Hunter, 2010b). In the psychodynamic literature, just treating the symptom without addressing the cause is discussed as insufficient and frequently iatrogenic, as it can lead to unconscious substitution of a worse symptom.

Some mental health counselors employ hypnosis to discover causes; but instead of completing the vital third and fourth hypnotherapeutic objectives with a client in hypnosis, they often try to deal with those causes at a conscious level, and often needlessly keep clients in therapy for months or years! Cognitive-behavioral therapy is the most widely used psychological therapy technique or approach among psychologists and mental health counselors. However, by itself, CBT simply is not enough because the client only learns to cope with a problem rather than resolve it (Emmerson, 2003). CBT is predominantly a left brain, logical, coping skills approach (Zarren & Eimer, 2002).

Do you think the first three objectives are enough? If so, think again. Numerous smokers have seen both of us over the years after stopping smoking previously with hypnosis, only to backslide weeks or months after their initial success. For that reason, we need to consider the next objective. The fourth objective is to help the client reframe his/her current understanding of the causes of the problem discovered, and the effects of these causes on the client in the past and, more importantly, from the present moment going forward.

## Subconscious Relearning (or Reprogramming)

If a smoker successfully stops smoking through hypnosis, even after discovering and releasing the cause(s) of the habit, his/her subconscious beliefs still influence the outcomes. Clients who *believe* that they will start smoking again because of previous failures may indeed light up again if they fantasize doing so often enough. Recall that imagination and emotion are the language of the unconscious; the smoking habit is unconsciously controlled and habits are imprinted by repetition (Zarren & Eimer, 2002). One of the cardinal laws of hypnosis is the Law of Dominant Effect which states that when the will (or willpower) is in conflict with the imagination (or emotion), the imagination always wins. Therefore, in order to insure successful hypnotherapy outcomes, the client must *believe* that the results will be lasting; otherwise he/she may be vulnerable to backsliding.

We can use numerous client centered techniques to facilitate adult understanding at a subconscious level, which is where adult understanding meets childhood learning and emotions. In order to achieve lasting results, therapeutic "insight" must be emotionally based. Intellectual (or left brain) understanding is not sufficient. Once the subconscious mind *believes* that a problem is resolved, unencumbered by cause(s) previously discovered and emotionally released, the client is then free to become self-empowered and achieve the desired goal. We may then ask the client to *imagine* fulfillment of his/her goal, and give additional suggestions that enable him/her to *expect* lasting success.

After accomplishing the third objective (i.e., emotional release), we may guide the client back to his/her peaceful place and then ask them to verbalize his/her own relearning. Paraphrasing the client's words back in the form of suggestions and imagery can help to fix in place in the subconscious mind the client's subconscious relearning (or reprogramming).

Notice the arrow going in both directions between numbers 1 and 4 in Figure 1. Suggestions and imagery enhance and reinforce the subconscious relearning process. They become much more powerful once the subconscious has discovered and released the cause(s) of a problem. They can serve to fix in place, on an unconscious and emotive level, the cognitive restructuring that has taken place in the client's conscious mind.

## Additional Comments

The number and variety of hypnotic techniques keeps growing as new ones are invented and old ones are updated or modified. Some techniques are designed specifically to release a problem, while others are designed to discover the causes and/or facilitate subconscious relearning.

Students of Hunter's hypnotherapy courses learn to evaluate the efficacy of any hypnotic technique based on discerning which of the four hypnotherapy objectives it may accomplish. This provides a solid foundation for practicing multimodal client centered hypnosis and obtaining results without the necessity of asking opinions regarding someone else's technique. If the technique works without risk to the client, *use it*; but learn to understand which of the four hypnotherapy objective(s) the technique accomplishes.

While it is not necessary to know every technique ever invented, the competent master of the art of hypnotherapy should have both width and depth of training, as there is *no* technique that is effective enough to work for all of the people all of the time. Even regression is not appropriate for all clients all the time. Over the years, clients have occasionally told Hunter or one of his former students that another therapist failed to help them, and then claimed that failure was because they were unable or unwilling to respond to hypnosis. Many hypnotists use only one modality (or program) which they attempt to utilize with all or most of their clients. Such hypnotists often get "certified" in a one-week or two-week training program that is too short to adequately teach a multimodal approach to hypnotherapy. This problem became prevalent throughout the 1980s and 1990s, as interest in hypnosis became more widespread, with the popularity of three-day training programs.

One-week or two-week certification programs still appeal to prospective students wanting to take short cuts in their training. Because the use of suggestion and imagery alone will help some of the people some of the time, graduates of short certification programs who have marketing skills often earn good money. Like the hotel hypnosis seminar marketers, they work with enough people to provide some credible testimonials from those who respond to suggestion and imagery alone.

While hypnotists using their favorite programs do help some of the people some of the time, their success rates are often overstated. The authors wish that they would call themselves "hypnotists" rather than hypnotherapists, and refer resistant clients to competent hypnotherapists. The competent hypnotherapist can help most of the people most of the time by practicing diversified multimodal client centered hypnosis.

## When is Hypnotic Regression Therapy Appropriate?

Hypnotic regression therapy is ideally suited for clients who have a problem that has a core cause that originated in the client's past (usually childhood, but not always). This is obvious for some problems, such as a fear of flying (or other fears and anxieties). With other problems, we must be good listeners to ascertain whether or not HRT is appropriate. When the need for hypnotic regression is not obvious, we can use ideomotor response questions as a guide to help make a determination whether to use HRT, parts therapy or one of its variations (ego state therapy, voice dialogue, etc.), a different technique altogether or whether to refer the client to another professional.

We cover how to set up ideomotor finger signals and how to use them in Chapter 3. For an in-depth treatment of ideomotor response questioning in hypnoanalysis beyond what this book covers, the reader is referred to Dabney Ewin and Bruce Eimer's *Ideomotor Signals for Rapid Hypnoanalysis: A How-To Manual* (2006). This topic is also presented in detail in chapter 6 of *The Art of Hypnotherapy* (Hunter, 2010b), as well as in chapter 3 of *Hypnosis for Inner Conflict Resolution* (Hunter, 2005).

## What Do We Look For?

When clients have a problem caused by past events that were painful emotionally and/or physically, there are usually a number of different causative incidents. However, with most clients, we normally look for only two events: the one that *caused* the problem and the one that *activated* the problem.

The event that caused the problem in the first place is called the initial sensitizing event (ISE), and we refer to the event that activated the problem as the activating event (AE). Note that some therapists and instructors label the activating event as the symptom producing event (SPE). There may be scores (or hundreds) of subsequent sensitizing events (SSE) that have compounded the problem over the years. However, if we effectively discover and release the ISE and the AE, the SSEs usually topple like dominos.

### Initial Sensitizing Event

When regression therapy is indicated, the client normally will have experienced an *initial sensitizing event* that is somehow emotionally connected to the presenting problem. The originating event (the ISE) sensitized the subconscious to a certain feeling, and the presenting problem is connected to that feeling. The ISE is often the same event that activated the problem, but not always.

If high emotion surrounds the presenting problem, the affect bridge technique (described in detail in Chapter 4) usually regresses the client right back to the ISE, because that is normally the first time the client experienced the same strong emotions that are connected to the problem. However, if the client suppresses the emotions attached to the problem, then we must employ other regression techniques to discover the ISE.

Often the initial sensitizing event has a direct and obvious connection to the presenting problem, such as a client with a fear of dogs that resulted from a vicious attack from a dog during childhood. However, numerous clients have an ISE that has no apparent connection to the presenting problem. In these instances, we usually have to uncover an activating event that happened days, weeks, months or even many years after the ISE.

Usually the ISE happens during childhood, but not always. Years ago, a hypnotherapy student had a fear of driving on the freeway. His ISE happened during an accident on the freeway, and it was the only event that required clearing with regression therapy.

Hypnosis historians may discover that Charles Tebbetts used the term "original sensitizing event" rather than initial sensitizing event. Roy Hunter chooses to use the latter term because it is more commonly recognized in the profession.

## Activating Event

The event that activates the problem is the *activating event*. As mentioned previously, some instructors refer to the event that triggers the problem as the symptom producing event (Banyan, 2005; Eastburn, 2007). The authors prefer to use the term AE for the activating event rather than SPE, although either term is correct. Although the activating event can be the same as the initial sensitizing event, it is not uncommon for the AE to take place during adolescence or adulthood rather than childhood.

To illustrate an example of an AE happening years after an ISE, a client with a fear of flying regressed back to a time at age six when she felt like she was "suffocating" while being tormented by a cousin. The event had no apparent connection whatsoever to her problem. However, the activating event happened during extreme turbulence in a commercial plane during her thirties. The window shade was fastened shut, and when asked about her feelings, she responded: "I feel like I'm suffocating, just as when I was six."

Note in the above example that there was no obvious connection of the ISE to the presenting problem; but the subconscious connected the dots during her AE, which activated the fear of flying.

## Subsequent Sensitizing Event

Events that cause further emotional and/or physical pain through the years can compound the severity of a client's problem. For example, an overweight child with low self-esteem who was emotionally abused by his parents could easily have his low self-esteem worsened because of bullying and/or name calling by schoolmates that he does not handle well.

Most clients do not need to have *subsequent sensitizing events* cleared when we properly discover and release the ISE and AE with HRT.

Unfortunately, however, some counselors and therapists not adequately trained to help clients with emotional release and subconscious relearning have used regression for "chaining back" through scores of SSEs over a period of many months. One of Roy's clients with a fear of birds actually found her phobia getting worse because of the combination of her psychotherapist chaining back and bringing her out of hypnosis at the first sign of abreactions (Hunter, 2010b). This resulted in her being re-traumatized repeatedly at a subconscious level, intensifying her fear of birds.

When the ISE and AE are properly discovered and released, appropriate ideomotor response questions can help determine whether it is necessary to look at an SSE as well. This procedure will be detailed in Chapters 4 and 5, along with numerous techniques for accomplishing the five phases of HRT. Note that some instructors refer to any SSE that follows the AE as a symptom intensifying event (SIE) (Eastburn, 2007). Again, the authors prefer to keep it simple, because often all the SSEs topple when both ISE and AE are discovered and released. When one or more SSEs remain and have to be cleared, the client's subconscious will normally let the hypnotherapist know, provided he/she has good rapport with the client and follows the procedures explained in Chapter 5 of this book.

### The Intake Evaluation

It is important to do a focused initial evaluation of your new client to gather information about the presenting problem along with relevant background information about the client. I (Eimer) routinely ask certain standard questions of every client as part of my initial interview. These questions comprise a "psychodynamic interview." The origins of this initial intake are discussed in detail in Ewin and Eimer (2006).

1. After gathering demographic information, which helps break the ice, I say to the client: **Tell me about your problem.** Many clients will answer this in a way that if taken literally describes the subconscious diagnosis. I then let the client talk and I listen and take notes.

2. My next question targets the origins of the problem. I ask: **When did it start?** If the client answers the question and gives a date, I ask: **What was going on in your life at that time?** If the client answers the initial "when did it start" question by talking about what was happening at the time, I take notes, ask clarifying questions and make sure to get some sort of date or time frame.

3. In line with our separation of ISEs, AEs and SSEs, I then ask, **When did it become a problem?** This is particularly important with incorrigible smoking and weight problems. How the client answers often gives useful insight into the motivation to stop, which can be enhanced and revivified in trance.

4. **What makes it better?** Aside from medicines, I note circumstances, times, dates and so on.

5. **What makes it worse?** If nothing makes it better or worse, I look for a near death experience. Nothing helps or hurts a person who is emotionally "dead."

6. **If you were cured, what would you do that you cannot do now?** This question addresses what things the symptoms or problem keep the client from doing, or what other problems they *seem* to solve. This is the issue of "secondary gain." If several things are mentioned, the *last* is the most important.

   Next, before I proceed to ask a bunch of more emotionally poignant questions, I ask the client: **What do you *like* for your friends to call you? May I call you that?** Then, I proceed to ask the questions, preceding each question with the client's preferred name.

7. *[Name],* **in your entire life** *[pause],* **what's the worst thing that ever happened to you?** This question pulls for helplessness. Helplessness leaves a highly emotional imprint, often causing symptoms.

8.  *[Name]*, **in your entire life** *[pause]*, **what's the worst thing you ever did?** This question pulls for the kinds of things that make the client feel guilty. Later, ideomotor questioning will ask if the presenting symptom is a form of self-punishment.

9.  *[Name]*, **in your entire life** *[pause]*, **what's the most frightened you've ever been?** This question pulls for trauma and also for experiences that might have led to the development of a phobia as protection against the same thing ever happening again.

10. *[Name]*, **in your entire life** *[pause]*, **what's the most angry you've ever been?** The emotional energy of anger is often *transduced* from fear or terror because we are often more comfortable with anger than fear. At least we can curse!

11. *[Name]*, **in your entire life** *[pause]*, **what's the most embarrassed you've ever been?** This question pulls for shame as opposed to guilt. Children are often cruel to each other. If a child limped, stuttered, was fat and so forth, an incident may have been devastating.

12. *[Name]*, **have you ever known anyone with the same or a similar problem?** Clients may model someone, usually one emotionally close and frequently dead. Keeping the symptom alive is a fantasy that the relationship is still alive.

13. *[Name]*, **what's the best thing that ever happened to you?** "Nothing" is the mark of severe depression. A healthy ongoing relationship is a useful predictor of a good outcome.

14. **If I had a magic wand, and one wish could come true, what would you wish:** "To get well" is ideal. After three tries, ask, **How many wishes would I have to give for you to wish to get well?** This question gives us some insight into strength of motivation.

15. **Is there anything else you think I ought to know?** This is the most important question of all. If the client answers it, *that is the*

*problem*. If the answer is "No," I hope you took good notes, because the subconscious is saying, "I already told you."

Additionally, I (Eimer) inquire about the client's medications, if any, and about the client's sleep, appetite, coping, mood, relationships, level of disability secondary to his/her presenting problems, the client's personal, educational and vocational history, previous therapies and treatments, surgeries, illnesses and medical, legal, psychiatric and substance abuse history.

Finally, as a psychologist, I (Eimer) assess and document the client's mental status, which includes the client's appearance, capacity to pay attention, language, speech, affect, mood, memory, comprehension, judgment, impulse control, thought content, any signs or symptoms of mental illness, mental stability, way of relating to examiner, level of insight, forthrightness and personality style.

# CHAPTER 2

# Guiding vs. Leading: The Risk of False Memories

Before even venturing into hypnotic regression, the therapist must understand the important difference between leading and guiding. Those who dare to facilitate regression without this vital understanding could find themselves on the wrong end of a lawsuit because of a pesky problem known as "false memory syndrome."

First of all, whenever a hypnotist or hypnotherapist helps a client attain a deep level of hypnosis, that client is *in rapport* with the hypnotist. If the level of trance is deep enough, that person may have an emotional desire to please the hypnotist and provide whatever answers are expected. In other words, if uninformed hypnotists or psychotherapists use hypnotic regression to *look for* past abuse, they may often find it where it never existed ... except in the imagination of client and/or therapist.

Second, the state of hypnosis is one of heightened suggestibility. Thus, a client who is in hypnosis is suggestible and sensitive to the demand characteristics that you set up consciously and unconsciously. Therefore, if you, the therapist, inadvertently or indirectly suggest that certain things might have happened, the hypnotized client is likely to take what you ask or say literally. This is because imagination is the language of the unconscious, and it accepts suggestions in a literal manner. Thus, you, the facilitator of the hypnotic regression, have to be careful about what you say and ask, as well as how you word your questions during your inquiry with the hypnotically regressed client.

Although Hunter's *The Art of Hypnotherapy* (2010b) devotes one lengthy chapter to hypnotic regression therapy, there are other books available that cover far more information than presented in that book.

Unfortunately, most books on hypnotic regression either empha-size past life regressions or they are heavy on case histories and light on techniques. However, two books worth reading are *Regression Hypnotherapy: Transcripts of Transformation* (Churchill, 2002) and *Transforming Therapy: A New Approach to Hypnotherapy* (Boyne, 1989). Another book, *Trance on Trial* (Scheflin & Shapiro, 1989), explains how inappropriate leading can occur during a hypnotic regression. Although the latter book discusses the forensic aspects of hypnosis, the warning applies to any hypnotherapist, psychologist or counselor employing hypnotic regression techniques: *avoid inappropriate leading*. If you do not heed that advice, you may find yourself in the middle of unwanted problems.

Seriously, the fact of the matter is that if you project your own pre-conceived opinions onto a client experiencing a hypnotic regression, you will taint the trance—and who knows the possible consequences? Read the words of Gordon Emmerson from his excellent book, *Ego State Therapy*:

> There is no way to distinguish a false memory from a real one. Hypnosis cannot distinguish these memories and Ego State Therapy cannot distinguish them. (Emmerson, 2003: 199)

Roy Hunter's own personal experience as a client validates Emmerson's opinion, as can be seen in the next section.

## Two Memories of the Same Event

After a local speaking engagement in the early 1990s, a hypnotist from the audience approached me (Hunter). She claimed that she was doing extensive research into explanations of the so-called "out of body" experiences (OBE) that children sometimes experience. She asked me to have lunch with her so that she could discuss her theories at length with me regarding alleged UFO abductions. Although I listened with an open mind, she raised my skepticism. Nonetheless, being an adven-turous soul, I agreed to allow her to hypnotize me as a participant in her research project. We will call her Linda (not her real name).

Before the hypnotic regression, I told her about my own OBE at age six after stepping on a scorpion. The closest doctor was 23 miles away, so he gave my parents instructions by telephone (I will spare you those details). By the time I went to bed on the evening of the day I was stung, the excruciating, spreading pain caused by the poisonous sting made my entire leg feel like it could explode. Later that night, my leg went totally numb; and then I saw a brilliant white globe of light hovering above my bed that appeared to be about the size of a basketball. Even at that young age, I marveled that the rest of the room was dark, reflecting none of the bright light. Then the numbness spread through my entire body and I was unable to feel anything or move anything. Furthermore, I could not look away from the light, so I tried to yell out to my sister who was sleeping nearby.

Not only was I unable to open my mouth, but I realized that I was no longer breathing! Then I started to float upward—and knew I was dying. With mental awareness only, I cried out to God reminding Him that I was only six years old and was too young to die just yet. Following that short silent prayer, I experienced the sensation of being slammed back into my body; and I cried out to my sister, who told me that I was only dreaming.

The next night, a similar globe of light hovered above my foot, but it was only the size of a baseball. This time the light did not frighten me because I was able to move. Also, somehow this globe of light gave me a mental or telepathic feeling that it was my guardian angel, and that it was there to look in on me. Within minutes, I fell asleep; and my foot was better the next morning.

Armed with only the information about the first night (but not the second night), Linda hypnotized me to medium depth, and employed regression to the specific event. She took me back to the moment when I first saw the bright light. She asked me to describe the room and my feelings, which I did. She then said, "I want you to go through the light and tell me if the light is a flying saucer. Were you taken into a spaceship?" (I have often told my students that the only thing missing in this regression was *X-Files* background music.) She proceeded to ask me one leading question after another, inappropriately leading me into "validating" her preconceived opinions, with me allegedly orbiting the earth for an hour or more during a UFO abduction experience. Additionally, she asked me if the aliens were short and gray, with black slanted eyes ...

When the session ended, I told her that my regression was fantasy caused by inappropriate leading. Linda's response was to tell me that my mind had repressed those memories, and that most of her subjects reported similar experiences. Does anyone wonder why?

As an experienced hypnotherapy instructor, it is very easy for me to assume that what emerged during that regression was false memory, especially in light of the blatant leading. For the next two years, I simply accepted the experience as a "false memory" (other than what was remembered by me at a conscious level prior to the regression). Eventually a competent hypnotherapist regressed me back to the same childhood event. Here is a summary of how that second regression unfolded.

When my body was paralyzed and I prayed inside my mind, the bright light told me that he was the death angel; but he told me it was not my time to die because I had something important to do. There was nothing that apparently happened between the time I felt myself starting to float up and the time that I was slammed back into my body—*no abduction*. The next day my leg was still swollen and in pain. That next night, however, when the globe of light hovered above my foot, it apparently spoke to me and said, "I am your guardian angel, and I'm here to complete the healing of your foot." I awoke the next day healed.

Here is what I tell my students about the above conflicting regressions. They both seem equally true, and they both seem equally fantasized, except for what I consciously remembered prior to the first regression. Professionally speaking, I believe that the mishandled regression gave me false memories. However, the second regression may be just as fictional as the first one, because *a client can create his/her own false memories in order to "prove" a point to someone, including himself!*

Please note the importance of my last statement. My own spiritual beliefs could easily have resulted in my subconscious mind creating false memories on the second regression, in order to disprove the first regression. Since both of these perceptions of the same event cannot be true, perhaps the truth might be a combination of the two regressions. Many hypnotherapists sitting in my workshops have offered to facilitate a third regression to help me identify the *real* memories; but there is a gift in my having two sets of memories for the same event. I can look my students and fellow professionals straight in the eye and teach something emphatically from my own experience: *If you are on the receiving end of a mishandled regression, you may not be able to distinguish fact from fantasy.*

Can I discover the truth of that OBE that happened when I was only six? In my opinion, the answer is *yes*. I would have to implement an investigation in order to obtain real world evidence to corroborate my perceptions. However, this experience serves as a constant reminder for me to emphasize the important difference between leading and guiding when facilitating hypnotic regressions and when teaching hypnotic regression therapy.

If you have preconceived opinions about the cause(s) of someone's problems while facilitating regressions, please set aside all those thoughts. Whether you base your opinions on professional, analytical or diagnostic skills, spiritual or religious beliefs, intuition or "psychic" awareness, you may drive your client farther from resolution if your opinions are in error. Ask open-ended questions that do not lead the client and be prepared to deal with what emerges. Also, be prepared to handle abreactions when clients remember their perceptions of emotional experiences. Make certain that the perceptions come from the client's inner mind and not from your own opinions.

While there is much more that we could write regarding how to inadvertently generate false memories during hypnotic regression therapy, our purpose here has been to share my (Hunter's) personal experience so that others may read and heed. Merely reading about the dos and don'ts of conducting regressions is often not enough to illustrate how false memoires can be created or confabulated.

Competent HRT can be far more valuable than hypnotic suggestion alone in helping clients release and reframe the causes of problems, and can help bring permanent resolutions. For me (Hunter) personally, all of the hypnotic regressions that I have experienced in *deep* hypnosis as a client have helped me, except for the "UFO abduction" described above.

Bruce and I recommend that hypnotherapy students invest in competent training before facilitating regressions; and if you are not yet comfortable with hypnotic regression therapy, add some width and depth to your training when possible. I hope that by the time you finish this book, you will respect the importance of avoiding inappropriate leading as well as facilitating client centered HRT.

## Inappropriate Leading vs. Appropriate Guiding

The best way to avoid inappropriate leading is to stick to asking "W" questions: who, what, when, where, why and how (how ends in "w"). When we ask questions that can be answered with a "yes" or "no" response, as we do when we use ideomotor finger signaling, we must be especially careful to avoid leading forced choices.

For example, the second author (Eimer) was conducting an HRT session with ideomotor signaling to help a client stop a two-pack-a-day smoking habit. She was regressed to what he mistakenly thought was the ISE for her smoking problem (i.e., not being able to stop smoking). She was a ten-year-old being told by her father who smoked that she should never start, because "once you start, you'll never be able to quit." Bruce asked her to answer with her fingers and her feelings, "Is this when you first get the idea that if you ever start smoking you'll never be able to quit?" The answer was "yes." However, he had made a mistake because he was inadvertently suggesting to her that she had this idea, but this was *his* hypothesis, not something the client had told him.

They worked on releasing this idea and reframing it, but the client starting smoking again. In a subsequent HRT session, in a regression to the time right before she had her first cigarette (age 13), the client verbalized that she did *not* believe she would be unable to stop if she started smoking, especially since smoking made her cough and gag; and her father had stopped and started again many times. Therefore, providing leading forced choices can result in false conclusions.

As another example, a well-known author years ago asked a volunteer during a hypnosis demonstration at a national hypnosis convention the following question: "Have you ever been influenced by an entity?" The volunteer moved the "yes" finger. Since many people would rather blame the devil instead of taking responsibility for their own mistakes, the subconscious can easily confabulate a real or imagined entity.

Roy Hunter provides a handout to his students containing the following examples of undesirable leading questions:

1. Does Daddy spank you now?
2. Does Daddy touch your private parts?
3. Go back to a past life when you starved to death.
4. Tell me if the light is a flying saucer.
5. Were you ever abducted by a UFO?
6. Go back to a time when you first felt a demonic presence.

Here are the histories behind each inappropriate leading question.

The first question occurred during a critiqued regression in Roy's classroom. The student client regressed back to a time when he said, "Daddy is punishing me." The student therapist then asked, "Does Daddy spank you now?" Instead of fantasizing a spanking, the student client immediately responded by saying that he was sent to his bedroom and grounded for the weekend, because the volunteer fortunately had retained a vivid memory of the event at a conscious level over the years. Nonetheless, that leading question could have resulted in a false memory if that event was not easily accessible to the conscious mind.

The second question was disclosed by a client seeing Roy for weight management. During the first few minutes of the intake, she told Roy that a family marriage therapist had helped her a year earlier for a family issue, and then offered her services when she stated that she wanted hypnosis for weight loss. Unfortunately, that therapist told her that childhood abuse was the usual cause for obesity; and the therapist then used hypnosis to regress her back to a time when her father hugged her. During that regression, the therapist asked, "Does Daddy touch your private parts?" Roy's client said that it took both her mother and two sisters over two weeks to convince her that her father never molested her.

The third example occurred when one of Roy's clients saw a hypnotist in Seattle who put her into hypnosis and said, "Go back to a past life when you starved to death." She told Roy that she immediately brought herself up out of hypnosis and told that facilitator that she did not believe in past lives.

The fourth example happened to Roy, and discussed above.

The fifth example happened at a national hypnosis convention when a published author hypnotized a volunteer and asked, "Were you ever abducted by a UFO?" To this day, Roy believes that the resulting regression may have been a total fantasy brought on by both the facilitator's convictions and the volunteer's beliefs in aliens. Even if there were a shred of truth in that regression, wouldn't it have been better if the facilitator had asked guiding questions instead of leading questions?

Roy Hunter witnessed the sixth example at a local demonstration, and he confronted the facilitator after the blown regression. Although the facilitator put on a good show with the client, Roy saw that same client several days later because she felt extreme guilt after having an alleged entity cast out of her in front of several dozen of her peers. When calling out the "Higher Power" part of the client, Roy asked, "What words of wisdom do you have for her?" The client's Higher Power part stated that the alleged entity was *not* hers, but instead claimed that it was an entity that followed the facilitator around in order to put on a good show. Roy confronted the presenter, who admitted that he was influenced to use hypnosis to look for entities after reading Edith Fiore's book, *The Unquiet Dead: A Psychologist Treats Spirit Possession* (1995).

The following section, a case history taken verbatim from Chapter 7 of *The Art of Hypnotherapy* (Hunter, 2010b), has several traps that an unwary hypnotherapist could have easily fallen into.

### Misplaced Money

After induction and deepening, I (Hunter) regressed the client back to the specific event that he described to me during the pre-induction interview (notice all the "W" questions).

> **RH:** Now go back to when you are sitting on the bed holding the money in your hand ... Which hand are you holding the money in? *[This leading question was appropriate here, because my objective was to lead him back to his last conscious memory of holding the money in his hand.]*
>
> **Client:** Right hand.
>
> **RH:** What are you doing with it?
>
> **Client:** I'm counting it.
>
> **RH:** What happens when you finish counting it?
>
> **Client:** I put it in a bag.
>
> *Client goes on to describe putting money under pillow and going to sleep.*
>
> **RH:** Move forward in time to when you first awaken ... What happens?
>
> **Client:** The phone rings. It's Johnnie, and I want him to call me later ... *[Client pauses]* I'm half asleep. I have to go to the bathroom ... *[Client pauses again]* But I need to do something with the money.
>
> **RH:** What do you do now?
>
> **Client:** I take the money with me ...

*Client describes holding the money while going to the bathroom, and is now standing at the door.*

**RH:** You're at the door now. What happens next?

**Client:** I step outside the back door and hide the money under the siding of the house.

*Note: If I had ended the session here, it would have been a mistake! What would you have done at this point? After a long pause, I break the silence.*

**RH:** You just put the money under the siding. NOW ... What are you doing?

**Client:** I'm standing back a few feet, looking to see whether or not it's visible.

**RH:** What do you think?

**Client:** Someone could find it here. I'd better hide it somewhere else ... I know! I'll look for a place near the garbage can ... *[Client pauses]* The money is in my hand again, and I'm looking at the garbage can ... I look under the lid. I'll move the can. Hmmm ... *[Long pause]* Perhaps this isn't a good hiding place. I just want to FORGET about this and go to bed with my girlfriend.

*Note: He was probably in a hypnotic trance state at the time he wanted to "forget" and go to bed, so his subconscious accepted the autosuggestion—and made him forget!*

**RH:** Where is the money now?

**Client:** I'm still holding it in my hand. I need a better place to hide it. There are some rafters in the basement—I think I'll go into the basement ... *[Long pause]*

**RH:** What do you decide to do?

**Client:** I'm going down the stairs now ... *[Another pause]* I'll open the basement door, and ... *[Client opens his eyes and shouts excitedly]* I KNOW WHERE IT IS!

Can you see where there were some traps that could have prevented this from being a successful session? My client had absolutely no memory (prior to hypnosis) of any of the events described after his last conscious memory of holding the money while sitting on the bed—not even the ringing phone. What if I had asked him if he hid it in the bathroom? How easy would it have been to assume that he'd left the money under the siding? What if I had concluded that he hid the money near the trash can? What if I had asked him if he threw the money away? Worse yet, what if I had simply asked him if he had put it back under his pillow when he got in bed with his girlfriend? Might he have falsely accused her of stealing it? Would you have avoided all these pitfalls?

Whether the regression objective is simply to remember details of a forgotten event (as in forensic investigative hypnosis) or whether it is for emotional clearing, we must remember to ask non-leading questions that enable clients to tell us what happened according to *their own perceptions*—not ours! If we try to fill in the details, memories might easily become distorted from the truth, as should be evident to the reader by now.

If you go looking for something, you may easily find it even where it does not exist. The subconscious is fully capable of fantasizing, which is why the testimony of a witness in court could be thrown out if hypnosis was used to enhance or refresh the memories of a witness (Scheflin & Shapiro, 1989). Clients can fantasize such things as physical or sexual abuse, UFO abductions, past lives, "entities" or demonic influences and so on.

## Avoid Preconceived Opinions

By now, it should be apparent that we need to avoid preconceived opinions. However, not all false memories originate from mishandled regressions. A "UFO abductee wannabe" can easily confabulate a very convincing story (too many episodes of *X-Files*?). The subconscious may easily respond to the fantasy (or altered memory) just as though it was true. In short, *we deal with perceptions* quite often rather than with reality. During hypnotic regression therapy, we need to help the client *release* the past, whether fact, fiction or a combination of both.

If you employ HRT to discover the core cause of a problem, it is extremely important that both you and the client set aside any pre-conceived opinions regarding the cause of the problem; and instead, allow the client's subconscious to go where it needs to go.

## The Danger of False Memories is *Real*

During the 1980s and 1990s, many therapists and mental health counselors unwisely used "memory recovery" with their clients. Some subsequently found themselves on the wrong end of lawsuits filed by parents of adult children who accused them of abuse that allegedly never happened. The misuse of hypnotic regression spawned many books on the topic of false memories. One of the most famous comes from Elizabeth Loftus, a member of the psychology department of the University of Washington: *The Myth of Repressed Memory: False Memories* (Loftus & Ketcham, 1996). Paul Durbin (2001) has an article posted on his website regarding the dangers of false memories (the article cites the work of Loftus). It also includes references to a num-ber of books on this topic.

Other experts also warn against the risk of false memories if the hyp-notist or hypnotherapist uses hypnosis to validate a preconceived opinion. Marx Howell, an authority on forensic hypnosis (and per-sonal friend of one of the authors), has warned against inappropriate leading many times over the years (Howell, 2011). The reader will find numerous articles on Howell's website at www.marxhowell.com.

The risk of false memories is so real that many states have disallowed the use of any court testimony enhanced by hypnosis (Scheflin, 2012; Wester & Hammond, 2011). In other words, a court of law can reject the testimony of a witness who was hypnotized to remember import-ant information for that case (Scheflin & Shapiro, 1989; Wester & Hammond, 2011). Inappropriate leading even during HRT can have serious consequences (Durbin, 2001; Yapko, 1995).

The biggest trap that hypnosis practitioners can fall into when conducting hypnotic regression sessions is inappropriate leading of the client. This can occur when the clinician uses regression to validate preconceived opinions regarding the causes of the patient's problems, and in its worst incarnation, was a major cause of what had been called "false memory syndrome" (Brown, Scheflin & Hammond, 1998; Scheflin & Shapiro, 1989).

When a person truly is in hypnotic trance, he/she is suggestible. Therefore, during a regression, well intended clinician comments verbalized to express empathy (e.g., "that little boy must be feeling angry", "daddy is scaring you", "little girl wants to run away") or as an expression of preconceived opinions (e.g., "your daddy needs you because mommy isn't giving daddy any attention"), can be accepted uncritically by the patient's unconscious and become imprinted suggestions. Such inappropriate leading comments can inadvertently result in the creation of false memories in that the patient acquires beliefs that something happened, that he or she felt a certain way, or that something happened for a particular reason, when in fact, such beliefs are not factually grounded. While the outcomes of inappropriate leading can be innocuous, they can also imprint suggestions that can go on to upset family homeostasis and ruin lives. In forensic and investigative hypnosis, inappropriate leading during hypnotic interviews can contaminate memories and result in a witness's testimony being ruled inadmissible in court (Scheflin, 2012; Scheflin & Shapiro, 1989; Brown, Scheflin & Hammond, 1998; Wester & Hammond, 2011).

The competent hypnotherapist who practices hypnotic regression therapy, and the competent forensic hypnotist, know the difference between guiding and inappropriately leading the patient and client respectively (Ewin & Eimer, 2006; Scheflin, 2012; Scheflin & Shapiro, 1989). Inappropriate leading can be avoided by asking open ended questions and through the appropriate use of ideomotor signals (Ewin & Eimer, 2006). It can also be avoided by conducting a good hypnosis pre-talk in which the limitations of hypnosis as a memory refreshment tool and the necessity of neutrality on the part of the hypnotist are discussed.

Competent hypnotic regression therapy has helped countless clients over the years. However, before using the technique it is imperative to understand how to properly employ HRT. The next five chapters discuss each of the five phases of hypnotic regression therapy in depth.

# CHAPTER 3

# Phase 1: Client Preparation

The preparation phase of regression therapy is just as important as the regression itself; because without it, we might not attain the desired results.

First, let us realize that hypnosis will not guarantee client veracity; so sufficient rapport and trust must be built during the previous sessions and/or the pre-induction interview to make it as easy as possible for the client to tell the truth. The client must also be educated as to what to expect during the hypnotherapy session, and what is expected of him or her. When we adequately accomplish the above, we may improve the probability of success by following these six steps of preparation:

1. Give a good pre-induction discussion.
2. Choose and use an appropriate hypnotic induction for client.
3. Deepen to at least medium depth, using convincers if necessary.
4. Establish (or confirm) peaceful place.
5. Establish (or confirm) ideomotor response signals (Steps 4 and 5 may be reversed if desired).
6. Verify hypnotic depth.

## Give a Good Pre-Induction Discussion

Because of the risk of false memories, we should always give a brief discussion about the risk of false memories before initiating a regression. This is because memories are stored on the basis of perceptions and are subject to distortions (Yapko, 1995).

### Seven Points to Consider in the Hypnotic Regression Therapy Pre-Talk

Consider including some or all of the following information in your pre-induction discussion before the client's first regression, even if he/she has experienced numerous previous hypnosis sessions. Put it into your own words.

1. Ask the client if he/she has either heard or read anything about false memories. (Over 90% of Roy's clients say "yes" in the Pacific Northwest of the U.S.A. and over 70% of Bruce's clients say "yes" in Pennsylvania.) Regardless of how the client answers, explain that the mind does not always remember things accurately, especially when emotions are involved. We can recall selected fragments of an experience and embellish them or combine them with other memories.

   For example, two children can witness a fight at school and give different versions of the same event just minutes after it happens. We frequently do not remember emotional events with total accuracy, because emotions often alter our perceptions. In other words, we remember events *according to our perceptions*, which may be fact, fantasy or a combination of both. In clinical, as opposed to forensic hypnosis, our objective is neither to prove nor disprove whether the client's perceptions are valid memories or fantasies, because we all typically respond to subconscious perceptions as though they are real. For example, a person with a fear of elevators responds to the perceived danger even if the logical mind knows that an elevator is safe.

2. Explain that the imagination is a valuable asset for experiencing a good regression, as the client will reap greater benefit from reliving (or revivifying) past experiences in the imagination rather than from simply remembering. Roy Hunter tells clients that in the imagination there is only the *now*. Whether we are fantasizing tomorrow, remembering yesterday or thinking about today, our subconscious minds will react as though our fantasy is happening in the *here and now*—whether it is fact, fantasy or a combination of both. In that sense, the imagination is like a time machine, allowing one to relive the past, reframe the past or create a desired future with as many of the five senses as desired. (For someone who loves *Star Trek*, we might say that the imagination is the holodeck of the mind.)

3. It is useful to remind the client that the information he/she reveals to the therapist is privileged and confidential. This helps facilitate the client's comfort with the idea of revealing personal perceptions and memories about his/her past.

4. If the client is inquisitive about the regression process itself, we can explain that the first objective is to discover the underlying perception or belief that caused (and might be maintaining) the problem; and that afterwards we will use hypnotic techniques to facilitate emotional release as well as new understanding (relearning) at a subconscious level, both of which are required for emotional healing.

5. Since the perceptions of details of the past may often differ from reality, one should carefully consider any potential consequences of laying blame on others for a client's presenting problem. Some clients may even respond to *guiding* questions with distorted memories of painful events; but if the client's goal is *release* and *relearning* rather than attributing blame, it may not be necessary to distinguish false memories from real ones. If release and relearning can take place, the client can still become empowered.

6. In light of the above, the client must indicate a willingness to release the past and heal, or we might consider declining to initiate a regression—and instead recommend that they see a family counselor or psychologist. Remember that we cannot force someone to change; so if we encounter conscious resistance in advance of the trance, suggest other professional help. Also, Roy often heard Charles Tebbetts tell clients before hypnotizing them in the classroom: "You could resist if you wanted to, but that's not why you're here"

7. Before inducing hypnosis, we might also recommend that the client set aside any preconceived opinions about the cause, and allow the subconscious to go where it needs to go. Remember the warning from Gordon Emmerson mentioned in an earlier chapter: if *either* the hypnotherapist *or* the client has a preconceived opinion

regarding the cause of a problem, it is often inaccurate (Emmerson, 2003).

These seven points are intended for discussion prior to employing HRT for the first time with a client, regardless of the number of previous sessions. If this is the client's very first hypnosis session with you, then consider the next section.

What to say is in **bold type**, while instructions are in *italics*. Pause briefly at an ellipsis (...).

### Bruce Eimer's Pre-Hypnosis Talk before the Client's First Induction

Before doing hypnosis with a client for the first time, it is essential that you conduct a pre-hypnosis talk in order to clarify and correct misconceptions about what hypnosis is, and to address and alleviate any fears that the client has about being hypnotized. Anxiety and fear about you or hypnosis will prevent your client from entering hypnosis or going deep enough to do effective regression work.

It is important to avoid following any scripts for this. Individualize your pre-hypnosis talk to the client and convey the information you cover in your own words. I (Eimer) typically cover the following areas in my pre-hypnosis talk:

1.  The three-part model of the mind: conscious, subconscious and unconscious.

2.  The fact that hypnosis is a natural altered state phenomenon and that we all enter and exit hypnoidal and hypnotic states naturally every day.

3.  The fact that clinical or therapeutic hypnosis is different from stage hypnosis.

4.  The fact that the power to enter hypnosis and to become suggestible (i.e., receptive to suggestions for change) lies within the client.

5. That no one can be made to do something they find objectionable with hypnosis, and that hypnosis is not a truth serum.

6. The fact that all hypnosis is self-hypnosis, the therapist is just a facilitator; and that anyone who wants to be hypnotized can experience hypnosis as long as they can focus and sustain their attention, and as long as they are not afraid and are partners in the hypnotherapy process. The client is told that they can resist if they want to, but then the therapist cannot be of help.

7. That hypnosis feels good. As used clinically, it is a state of relaxed effortless attention, increased suggestibility and controlled day-dreaming and imagination. That anyone who can daydream can do hypnosis, and that the client should simply think and imagine the things that the therapist suggests as long as these things are acceptable. In addition, if the therapist says anything that does not feel right, the client can either ignore it or change it in his/her own mind to what he/she wants and needs to hear.

8. If you use touch as part of your hypnotherapy techniques, it is important to explain where and why you touch clients during the hypnosis and hypnotherapy process and why you do so (e.g., hand, arm, shoulder, head, forehead). *You must always get permission to touch your client.* If your client does not want to be touched, or if touch is contra-indicated, *you must not touch your client.*

After conducting your intake evaluation (as explained in Chapter 2), doing your pre-hypnosis talk and assessing your client's readiness to enter hypnosis, you must ask your client for permission to do hyp-nosis. In addition, as emphasized above, you must always ask for the client's permission to touch them if you need to use touch as part of your hypnosis and hypnotherapy procedures. I like to word this as Cal Banyan teaches in his classes (www.CalBanyan.com). I ask the client:

> **Would you like to do hypnosis with me now?**
>
> **Is it all right for me to touch your hand, your arm, your shoulder and even maybe your head or forehead?**

Again, if the client does not wish to be touched, avoid all touch techniques. Also, if you forget to ask permission prior to the induction, do not employ touch techniques.

Now let us discuss the remaining steps of the HRT preparation phase.

## Choose and Use an Appropriate Hypnotic Induction for the Client

The best induction for most of your clients most of the time is *the one you like best*. Your confidence and competence with your favorite induction will come across subconsciously, and most willing clients will respond provided you have a good rapport. Nonetheless, no induction works with all the people all the time, so master several alternate inductions.

Mental confusion techniques often work well with analytical clients (Hunter, 2010a). If your client has a short attention span, you may wish to use either a rapid induction or one that is fairly quick. Therefore, even though most clients will respond to your favorite induction, it is wise to learn at least one mental confusion induction and one fast induction.

For your convenience, several induction techniques and scripts appear in the last section of this chapter, which also include other steps of the preparation phase.

## Deepen to Medium Depth, Using Convincers if Necessary

Be patient and persistent, taking sufficient time to deepen a client appropriately. If your client is an analytical resister, an insufficient trance depth may result in either an unsuccessful regression or one that has only temporary or partial results. This fact has been brought home to both of us over the years. We have both conducted our fair share of failed regression sessions because of insufficient trance depth.

While the techniques presented in subsequent sections of this chapter offer some deepeners and convincers, be sure to use other resources if needed in order to master a variety of techniques that help deepen the trance state.

## Establish or Confirm the Client's Peaceful Place

If we have already established a peaceful place (or safe place) in a previous session, we may simply guide the client back there and ask him/her to confirm being there; otherwise, it is important to help the client establish a peaceful place because client centered HRT involves the peaceful place at least twice in every regression.

Although it is permissible to ask the client in advance of the trance to describe his/her ideal place of peace, occasionally a client chooses a different place during hypnosis. Here is a sample script that allows the client to choose a safe or peaceful place during hypnosis.

> Now, imagine an ideal, peaceful place. A place that is ideally peaceful for you. Your imagination is your own private rehearsal room of your mind. You CAN DO ANYTHING you want, or BE ANYWHERE you desire. So, just choose a safe, peaceful place, and IMAGINE that you are there in your peaceful place right now ...
>
> Imagine sights, sounds and feelings that are SO peaceful, SO serene and SO relaxing ... that it is as though you are becoming a part of the tranquility that you imagine. That there is an INNER PEACE just flowing through every part of your being ... physically, mentally, spiritually and emotionally.
>
> Now, as you imagine an ideal place of peace, a place that is ideal for you, touch your thumb to a finger that you choose as your peaceful place finger ... and now take a deep breath and think the word, "RELAX" ...
>
> Anytime you touch your thumb to your peaceful place finger or you take a deep breath and think the word "RELAX," you connect to your place of peace ... and any time I ask you to go to your peaceful place, go there immediately.
>
> *Give other suggestions as appropriate.*

## Establish or Confirm Ideomotor Response Signals

There are two reasons for this step of the preparation phase. First of all, finger response signals help determine *trance depth* in the last step of the preparation phase. More importantly, we use ideomotor response questions in the regression session itself to *confirm emotional release* and to determine whether additional regressions are necessary to discover any additional events, whether for an ISE, AE or SSE.

We should help the client establish a finger response for "yes," "no," and "I don't know" or "I'm not ready to answer yet." The third response increases the probability that any yes or no responses are more accurate, because the subconscious can lie if there is an emotional desire to cover up the cause (Hunter, 2010b).

Even if we have already established finger response signals in a previous session with a client, we should still confirm the same signals for the current session. Although it is very rare for a client to change a previously established finger response, occasionally clients of each of the authors have done so.

Two methods of establishing ideomotor response signals appear below. The combined experience of decades demonstrates that you may use either of the procedures and still obtain results, or you may edit either script to your liking as long as it gets results.

### Bruce Eimer's Procedure for Establishing Ideomotor Response Signals

The procedure that Bruce Eimer employs was developed by Dabney Ewin, and has been previously described in Ewin and Eimer (2006).

> I am going to teach you a way to signal how you feel without even talking—please close your eyes.
>
> SETTING UP "YES": You know that if we were just having a conversation, and I asked "Is your name [*say client's name*], you could simply nod your head up and down without talking, and I

would know you were saying "yes." If I ask you a question, and you feel the answer is "YES"—you have a "yes" feeling about it, you agree—this finger *[Lift client's index finger slowly as this is said]* will slowly rise to signal that you agree, that it feels okay, that it feels "yes."

TEST QUESTION: Do you like for your friends to call you *[name]*? That's right. *[Gently pushing index finger back down]* Of course, you've already told me that you like for your friends to call you *[name]*.

DEEPENER: Every time your feelings answer a question, you'll go deeper and deeper and get more in touch with your deepest and most heartfelt feelings.

SETTING UP "NO": If I ask you a question and you disagree— you have a "no" feeling about it, it just doesn't feel right—this finger *[Gently lift client's middle finger]* will slowly rise to signal that you disagree. You don't have to know why, it just doesn't feel right, the answer is "no." *[Now ask a question you know is "no."]*

SETTING UP "I DON'T KNOW" OR "I'M NOT READY TO ANSWER": If I should ask a question and you don't know the answer, OR you're not ready to answer YET or you don't want to answer, just signal with your thumb *[Gently lift client's thumb]*, and that's all right.

SETTING UP "NEED TO TALK": And if something crosses your mind that you want to tell me or you want to ask a question, just raise your hand *[Gently lift the client's hand and let it fall back]* and we'll talk.

*[If the client raises their hand during the session, say]* "SPEAK to me and tell me what's on your mind."

SEALING THE CONTRACT: Now, my first question to your feeling mind is, and please answer with your fingers, with your feelings, yes or no, is it all right for me to help you with this problem?

## Roy Hunter's Procedure for Establishing Ideomotor Response Signals

I (Hunter) created this procedure in 1984, and simply ask the client's subconscious to choose the appropriate finger or thumb representing the "yes" and "no" responses, as well as the "I don't know" or "I'm not ready to answer" response.

> **I'm going to ask a series of questions that can be answered YES or NO, and would like for you to allow the response to come from your subconscious or your inner mind. If I ask you a question, and the answer feels YES, you agree, please indicate with a finger that you choose to indicate "yes," and move that finger now.** [*Make a note of it.*] **If I ask you a question, and the answer feels NO, you do not agree, choose a different finger or thumb and indicate the "no" response now.** [*Note it.*] **And if I ask you a question, and the answer either feels "I don't know" or "I'm not ready to answer yet," just raise a different finger or thumb, and indicate that response now.**

Although my method is not nearly as thorough as Bruce Eimer's procedure, both methods have passed the test of time. Use the one you prefer.

## Verify Hypnotic Depth

When a client makes it obvious that he/she has attained a somnambulistic level of hypnosis, we may guide the client right into a regression with an appropriate regression technique. More often than not, however, it is necessary to verify the client's hypnotic depth.

The technique that Roy Hunter uses is a variation on a technique taught to him during the 1980s by Sean Longacre, which enables the subconscious to provide feedback that helps to estimate the client's hypnotic depth.

Many people consciously underestimate their own trance depth (including experienced hypnotherapists), but finger responses often indicate either lighter or deeper levels than the client might claim verbally. Here is a script that closely resembles what Hunter teaches to hypnosis professionals.

> **Now, imagine a scale of 100 to the number 1. The number 100 represents being awake but with your eyes closed, while the number 1 is absolutely as deep as you can go in hypnosis without falling asleep. The number 50 is halfway there. If you are 50 or deeper, please indicate by moving the "yes" finger ...**
>
> *If "yes" continue to assess your client's trance depth. If "no" or "I don't know," then deepen until your client indicates "yes." (Note that the above statement is an* appropriate *leading suggestion, designed to lead the client into a state of hypnosis deeper than 50. Inappropriate leading is when a client responds to leading questions or suggestions that lead him/her into assumptions that could result in fantasy of past events or false memories.) Once your client signals that he/she is at a 50 or deeper, ask:*
>
> **Are you 40 or deeper?**
>
> *If "yes," continue to assess your client's trance depth. If "no," then deepen until the client is deeper than 40. Then ask:*
>
> **Are you 30 or deeper?**
>
> *At this point, regardless of the client's response, ask:*
>
> **Are you deep enough to continue into the next phase of this session?**
>
> *If the answer is "no" to the above question, go back to deepening before continuing into the next phase of HRT. If the answer is "yes," proceed with the regression technique of choice. If it is necessary to deepen further, do so and then repeat the above question until you receive a "yes" response. Then say:*
>
> **Thank you. Now that you are deep enough, we will proceed with the next phase of this session ...**

Recognize that depth of hypnosis is a metaphoric label for level of sug-gestibility; and level of suggestibility is also associated with the believ-ability of imaginings. The more deeply absorbed in hypnotic trance a client is, the more suggestible the client becomes. This is when the critical factor of the mind relaxes and the client's subconscious is more receptive to suggestions, as long as they are worded in a manner that the subconscious can understand and accept.

In terms of the scale above, here are our clinical guidelines:

- Clients who are unable to get below 50 (after several deepening attempts) are not likely to be capable of revivifying memories in their imagination sufficiently to benefit from regression therapy until another session, unless we employ the affect bridge technique (because emotion puts the client into the right brain). Someone who suffers from "analysis paralysis" will often resist a beneficial regression by remembering rather than reliving (or revivifying) in the imagination. The analytical person in light trance may eas-ily neutralize whatever memories and accompanying emotions emerge from the inner mind. This conclusion comes from our own personal experiences as clients and clinicians, as well as the experi-ences of others reported to us in workshops.

  Once we conclude that a client will not go deep enough for regres-sion during a hypnosis session, we change gears. We can give the client suggestions and imagery to resolve the problem, blended with post-hypnotic suggestions for attaining a deeper level of hyp-nosis at the next session.

- Some clients who indicate levels between 40 and 50 are able to experience a successful regression or parts therapy session, although it is usually best to make several attempts to get the cli-ent below 40 in order to have more favorable odds for a successful session.

- When responses verify depth levels between 40 and 30, the deci-sion to initiate regression should revolve around whether the client's subconscious believes that the hypnotic depth is sufficient to continue into the next part of the session. At depths of 30 or below, most clients accept suggestions that they are now deep enough.

Be aware that a small percentage of clients may ask you to continue deepening until they are too deep to respond verbally, simply because they feel very good going that deep. If a client goes too deep to respond verbally, we may suggest that he/she come up to a level of hypnosis that is still deep, but just high enough to speak verbally. We suggest the following:

> **As I count from 1 to 3, please come up to a level of hypnosis that is still deep, but just light enough for you to speak out loud. Allow yourself to find either your perfect level of trance, or your IDEAL depth ... and say "yes" when you are there.**

Once the client reaches sufficient trance depth, ask the subconscious to keep the client at his/her *ideal* depth (emphasize the word *ideal*), and to confirm that this suggestion is acceptable at all levels of consciousness by moving the "yes" finger. Wait for the response, repeating the above suggestions if necessary until you get the desired response. We are now ready to guide the client into a hypnotic regression.

Before moving on to that phase, however, we wish to offer some sample induction and deepening techniques with scripts.

## Induction Techniques

What follows are eight induction techniques—the first directive, the second naturalistic and permissive, and the third and fourth directive and permissive; the next two are mental confusion inductions; and the seventh is a rapid induction.

For a review of other available hypnotic induction and deepening techniques, refer to Zarren and Eimer's *Brief Cognitive Hypnosis* (2002), Eimer's *Hypnotize Yourself Out of Pain Now!* (2007), chapters 5 and 6 of

Hunter's *The Art of Hypnosis* (2010a) or any other credible basic hypnosis books.

Note that some of the sample scripts show the counting into hypnosis to be forwards, while others are counting the client down into hypnosis. Feel free to reverse the direction of counting according to your own preference, as most clients will respond regardless of which direction you count. That being said, Roy Hunter discovered from experience in 1983 that if you count forward to deepen the trance, that same client might go even deeper if the awakening count is in the same direction as the numbers used during the induction and deepening.

## Dave Elman's Method

Bruce's favorite directive induction technique is an adaptation of the Elman–Banyan Induction (Banyan & Kein, 2001; Elman, 1984) that he learned from Calvin Banyan at the intensive hypnosis and hypnotherapy course on Banyan's 5-PATH® Hypnosis and Hypnotherapy System. This induction is based on Dave Elman's original method (Elman, 1984). This Elman–Banyan Induction is brief, elegant, has built in measures of client cooperation and participation in the hypnosis process, and built in trance ratifiers, convincers and deepeners.

Here is the essence of the words I (Eimer) use:

*Begin by holding your hand horizontally about one to two feet in front of the client's eyes, palm facing the client and your fingers together. Verbalize the following as you slowly raise your hand slightly above the client's head and then slowly pass it downward.*

**Take a look at my hand, take in a nice deep breath** *[as your pass your hand upward],* **hold it for a moment, now let that breath out slowly** *[as you pass your hand downward],* **close your eyes, and relax deeply.**

*The following is a measure of client cooperation and participation:*

**Now shift your attention to your eyelids. You can relax your eyelids so much that they just won't work. Please do that now. Once you are sure that you have relaxed your eyelids so much**

that they just won't work, check to make sure that they won't work ...

*Watch your client and as long as the client does not open his/her eyes, reinforce him/her by saying:*

Very good. Now stop checking and go deeper relaxed. Now take the feeling of relaxation that you are allowing in your eyelids and move it into the top of your head. Relax the top of your head just as you let your eyelids relax. Now let that feeling of relaxation wash all the way down your body, all the way down into the bottoms of your feet, just like a warm wave of comforting relaxation. And with each and every breath that you exhale, and each and every word that I say, regardless of the meaning of my words, feel your body relaxing more and more and feel yourself going deeper into relaxation.

*The following is another measure of client cooperation and involvement as well as a deepening technique:*

Now, in a moment, with your permission, I am going to lift your arm by the wrist to check how well you have relaxed so far *[gently pat the client's wrist nearest you]*. So let that arm be completely relaxed and permit me to do ALL the lifting. And when I drop that arm back down, just let that arm drop. Let that arm be heavy and limp so that it just drops down, and just as that arm drops down all by itself, let yourself just drop way down into a deep sound state of relaxation *[gently lift client's arm and drop it]*. That's right. Just let it drop as you drop further down into deep relaxation.

*Note that this is Step 3 of the preparation phase if using HRT:*

Now let's double your relaxation. So, once again shift your attention to your eyelids and make sure that they are so relaxed that they just won't work. Test them to make sure that they won't work ... Good. Now stop testing and go twice as deep into relaxation as you spread the relaxation in your eyelids into the top of your head and then let that relaxation wash down your entire body into the bottoms of your feet ... Excellent.

Now let's do that again. Once again shift your attention to your eyelids and test them to make sure that they won't work ... Good. Now stop testing and go twice as deep into relaxation as you spread the relaxation in your eyelids into the top of your head and then let that relaxation wash down your entire body into the bottoms of your feet ... Excellent.

*The following is a covert suggestibility test for suggested amnesia:*

Now I am going to help you relax mentally. In a moment, I'm going to ask you to count out loud SOFTLY and SLOWLY starting with the number 1. And I'm going to ask you to let it be different from every time that you have ever counted in that, this time, you are going to put less and less effort into each successive number that you count. So that, after counting just a few numbers, you will be putting zero effort into the numbers and you will have relaxed the numbers out of your mind, and they will be gone. Want this and you will experience it. Now begin counting and put less and less effort into each number that you count as you just relax the numbers away. Let it happen and soon the numbers will be gone. And when the numbers are all gone, raise this index finger to signal that the numbers are all gone.

*Gently stroke the index finger of the client's hand closest to you. Wait for the client to begin counting and after the client says each number, the therapist says any combination of the following:*

SOFTER, SLOWER, with only half as much mental effort, doubling your relaxation.

*When the client raises their index finger, gently lower it and say:*

Good. Nothing, nothing, nothing. Now go deeper. Let yourself go deeper. You can always go deeper.

*If the client gets to 6, at 6 suggest to the client,* NOTHING, NOTHING, NOTHING *as you gently tap the client's index finger. Then keep saying the following until the client loses the numbers:*

SOFTER, SLOWER, with only half as much mental effort, doubling your relaxation.

*Now, to help your client further deepen his/her relaxation, say the following:*

Now I'd like you to listen as I count from 1 to 10. And as I count each number, let yourself go much deeper into relaxation and hypnosis so that you can feel much more comfortable. More and more comfortable and more and more deeply relaxed as I say each number ... and when I get to 10, you will be 10 times as deeply relaxed, and more relaxed than you have ever been. And as you go into deep relaxation and hypnosis, the doorway into your inner mind opens so that we can do the work that you are here to do. 1 ... relaxing further. 2 ... going deeper and deeper. 3, way, way, way more deep. 4, deeper and deeper with each and every breath you take. 5, attending only to the sound of my voice, and going deeper and deeper with each and every word I say regardless of the meaning of my words. 6 , and as you go deeper and deeper, you get more in touch with your deepest feeling mind. 7, into a deeper and sounder and more relaxed state. 8, way, way deeper, getting more in touch with the part of you that is most precious. 9, and as your body relaxes, your mind relaxes, and your body relaxes much further. And 10, ten times as deeply relaxed. With nothing to bother or disturb you, such that all you care about now is how much more deeply relaxed you can go.

*Administering the eye catalepsy test as a convincer to ratify and deepen the client's trance (Step 3 of the preparation phase of HRT):*

Now please shift your attention once again to your eyelids. And as you focus on the feeling in your eyelids, your eyelids become shut tighter. The more you focus on your eyelids the tighter they become. And as I count from 1 to 3, your eyelids will TWITCH and TIGHTEN. And when I get to 3, you will try to open them but you will not be able to.

*Lightly begin tapping with two fingers in the middle of the client's forehead right above the bridge of the nose.*

1, your eyelids are twitching and tightening and locking down tight. 2, your eyelids are shut tighter and tighter, locking down and stuck together like glue. 3, locked down tight, you try to open them but you cannot. Try to open them but you cannot. They are locked so tightly together, you try to open them but you cannot. GOOD. Now stop trying, relax and go deeper.

*Proceed to doing the therapy. When it is time to emerge your client up out of hypnosis (Step 2 of Phase 5 if using HRT), say:*

Okay. In a moment, I am going to count from 1 up to 5. And as I count up, you will comfortably emerge from hypnosis, and when I get to 5, and not before I say the number 5, you will open your eyes and emerge from hypnosis. And when you open your eyes, you will be wide awake, alert, refreshed and you will be sound in mind, sound in body and in control of your feelings. And you will feel really, really good.

*Count to 5 and when you reach 5, say:*

And you do feel good don't you ...?

## Joseph Barber's Naturalistic Method

Eimer's favorite indirect and naturalistic induction technique is inspired by Dr. Joseph Barber's permissive and conversational induction style. This is most famously exemplified in his relaxation induction of analgesia stairs script (Barber, 1996; Barber & Adrian, 1982). This permissive style of induction is often appropriate with more resistant clients, and in this author's opinion, is also very elegant.

Here is the essence of the words I (Eimer) use. Note the absence of any overt hypnotic challenges; convincers and trance ratification, however, are built in.

*Obtain client's permission to do hypnosis:*

Would you like to do hypnosis with me so that you can feel more comfortable and relaxed? Okay. Great. Then, why don't you find a position in which you can listen without much effort. And

I certainly want you to know that you can adjust your position at any time to get more comfortable ... That's great.

Now, when you are ready, I'd like to invite you to close your eyes comfortably without squeezing them tight, and please keep them comfortably closed until I ask you to open them, or until you want to open them ... Good. And now with your eyes closed, you can concentrate more easily on what I'm saying ...

Now, I'd like you to notice how much more comfortable you can feel by just taking one very big, satisfying, deep breath. Go ahead ... take a big, deep, satisfying breath ... And notice how good that feels ... And please feel free to take several more big, deep breaths, and notice if it feels more satisfying. Just notice ...

There is no need to try to make anything happen now. Simply give yourself permission to notice what you feel and how differently you can feel ... For example, how warm your neck and shoulders can feel ... And how relaxed your neck and shoulders can feel ... And how relaxed your back can feel ... And how limp and floppy your arms can feel ... And how relaxed your chest can feel ... And how soft your abdomen can feel ... That's right. And how loose and limp and lazy your legs can feel.

Now, I'd like to ask you simply to pay attention to your breathing. And I am asking you to pay attention to your breathing because it might help you to feel more relaxed. There is no need to try to change your breathing, or for that matter, to TRY to do anything at all. I'm just asking you, inviting you, to pay attention to your breathing because as you do, you may find that your breathing begins to change all by itself. Enjoy noticing how your breathing changes—perhaps it is becoming slower, more shallow, more comfortable and more relaxed ... That's right.

And with each and every natural and comfortable breath you take, I'd like you to notice how much more comfortable and relaxed you feel as you exhale ... Almost as if with each and every breath that you exhale, you are blowing stress and tension out into the atmosphere never to return ... And as you release more and more stress and tension with each breath you exhale, notice how you can just feel more and more relaxation sinking in, as you sink comfortably into that chair.

Good ... Now, as you continue breathing, easily and comfortably and rhythmically, all I'd like you to do now is to just picture in your mind ... just imagine, a staircase, any kind you like, with ten steps, and you at the top ... You can see that staircase any way you like ... and just notice yourself at the top of the staircase, and the step that you are on ... But however you see it is just fine ... And in a moment, but not yet, I'm going to begin to count, out loud, from 1 to 10 ...

And as you may have already guessed, as I count each number, I'd like you to take a step down that staircase, see yourself stepping down, feel yourself stepping down, one step for each number I count ... And all that you need to do is notice, just notice how much more comfortable and relaxed you can feel at each step, as you go down the staircase ... One step for each number that I count ... the larger the number, the further down the staircase, the further down the staircase, the more comfortable you can feel, and the more comfortable you feel, the more relaxed you will feel ... one step for each number ... All right, you can begin to get ready ... And now, I'm going to begin counting ...

1, one step down the staircase ... 2, two steps down the staircase ... Nice ... 3, three steps down the staircase ... And I wonder how much more relaxed you feel ... I wonder if there are places in your body that feel more relaxed than others ... Perhaps your shoulders feel more relaxed than your neck ... perhaps your legs feel more relaxed than your arms ... I don't know, and it really doesn't matter ... all that matters is that you feel comfortable ... that's all that matters ... 4, four steps down the staircase, perhaps feeling places in your body that are relaxing more than others ... 5, five steps down the staircase ... halfway down, and hopefully right now, really, really enjoying your experience of relaxation and comfort ... 6, six steps down the staircase ... perhaps you can notice that all the sounds you can hear are becoming a part of your experience of comfort and relaxation ... that anything you can notice becomes a part of your experience of comfort and relaxation ... 7, seven steps down that staircase ... that's fine ... 8, eight steps down the staircase ... perhaps noticing that as you relax more and more, your pulse rate is slowing down, your blood pressure is lowering, and your breathing is slower and more rhythmic and more regular ... and 9, nine steps down this staircase, breathing comfortably, slowly and deeply restful, perhaps noticing that the relaxation is really sinking in, the pleasant, restful, comfortable relaxation just spreading through your body ... And 10, ten steps down the staircase, all the way at the bottom of the staircase, feeling so pleasantly restful, and just continuing to notice the growing, spreading, comfortable relaxation ... and that there's nothing to bother you, and nothing to disturb you, as you enjoy being deeply and comfortably relaxed, and noticing perhaps the restful pleasantness as your body just seems to sink down, deeper and deeper into the chair, with nothing to bother, nothing to disturb ... as that chair holds you comfortably and warmly ... with nothing to bother and nothing to disturb you as you continue to feel more and more comfortable, more and more rested ... more and more comfortable ... DEEPLY, DEEPLY RELAXED ... deeper with every breath you take ... and deeper with each word that I say regardless of the meaning of my words.

*Post-hypnotic suggestions:*

And I wonder if you'll be pleased to notice that the things we talk about today, with your eyes closed, are the things which you'll remember tomorrow, and the next day ... and maybe even next week ... I wonder if you'll decide to let the memory of these things rest quietly in the back of your mind ... And I also wonder if you'll notice that you'll feel surprised that your visit here today is so much more pleasant and comfortable than you might have expected ...

*Now give a post-hypnotic suggestion for entering this state in the future whenever it is appropriate and safe for your client to do so:*

In fact, I wonder how pleased you will be to notice that today ... and any day, that whenever you feel your head resting back against a headrest or a pillow ... that whenever you feel your head resting back like this, and whenever it is appropriate, whenever you want to relax like this, and as long as it is appropriate to relax like this ... you'll feel reminded of how very comfortable you are feeling right now ... Perhaps even more comfortable than you feel right now ... comfortable and relaxed ... with nothing to bother and nothing to disturb.

*At this point, proceed to doing your therapeutic work.*

*Emerging the client (Step 2 of Phase 5 if using HRT):*

And in a moment, but not yet, not until you're ready, I'm going to count up from 1 to 10. And as you know, I'd like you to feel yourself going back up the steps and emerging from this hypnosis ... one step for each number ... and you'll have all the time you need ... because after all, time is relative ...

When I begin counting, feel yourself slowly and comfortably going back up the steps, one step for each number I count ... more and more alert as you go back up the steps, one step for each number I count ... and when I reach 8, your eyes will be almost ready to open ... when I reach 9, they will have opened ... and, when I reach 10, you'll be alert, awake, refreshed ... perhaps as though you've had a nice nap ... alert, refreshed and comfortable.

1, 2, 3 ... feel yourself going back up the steps ... getting ready to emerge, knowing that when you open your eyes you'll feel great. 4, 5, 6 ... more than halfway back up, more and more alert ... no rush, plenty of time ... feel yourself becoming more and more alert ... 7, 8, 9 ... almost all the way up ... your eyes opening ... And 10 ... alert, comfortable, refreshed, awake, feeling sound in mind and sound in body and in control of your feelings. And you do feel good don't you?

## Helen Watkins's Arm Drop Method

Another one of Eimer's favorite rapid and directive relatively permissive induction techniques is called the arm drop or reverse arm levitation technique that Eimer learned personally from the late Helen Watkins (Watkins & Watkins, 1997). This induction is often appropriate with resistant clients. It is also a great induction to use as a lead-in to doing regression work and as a method of regressing a client.

Here is the essence of the words I (Eimer) use. Note the absence of any overt hypnotic challenges; convincers and trance ratification, however, are built into the method. The regression method used is the Staircase of Time.

> *Position the client's right or left arm at a 45 degree angle upward with the back of the hand slightly above eye level. Then begin saying:*
>
> STARE at one of the fingers, either the INDEX or the MIDDLE finger. You may continue to LOOK at it or, if you wish, close your eyes and visualize it in your MIND'S EYE. As you fixate your gaze on that finger, you will notice that the other fingers tend to FADE OUT OF FOCUS and that your entire arm begins to feel HEAVIER and HEAVIER. The longer you CONCENTRATE on that finger the HEAVIER and HEAVIER your arm becomes, BUT you will NOT go into a state of DEEP RELAXATION until that arm has come ALL THE WAY DOWN.
>
> KEEP CONCENTRATING on that finger while the arm gets HEAVIER and HEAVIER. Notice that as the arm is getting heavier, it is slowly coming DOWN, DOWN, DOWN. But, you will NOT relax into a deep and profound state of relaxation until the arm is all the way down and touching. Going DOWN, DOWN, DOWN, DEEPER and DEEPER, DEEPER and DEEPER as you go down with it DEEPER and DEEPER.
>
> Good. Now imagine you and I are standing together at the top of a staircase. This is a very special staircase—a staircase back in time. Look down this staircase. Look back in time. There are ten steps down this staircase. Ten steps back in time. The steps

are covered with a soft, plush carpet of your favorite color. As you look further down this stairway back in time, the stairs seem to fade into a soft warm darkness. Now, we can walk down those stairs together. If that feels all right to you, your "yes" finger will rise to signal that it feels all right. *[Wait for ideomotor finger signal]*

Now, as you walk down these stairs, you can slide your hand along the smooth hardwood banister. And I will walk down with you if that's all right with you, and I will count the steps we walk down, starting with the top step which is step number 10. Each count downward is another step down the soft, plush carpeted stairs. And when we get to the bottom of the steps, you will be *[age regression:* **X years old;** *event regression:* **at your tenth birth-day party;** *symptom regression:* **right before the first time you had that headache]**.

Let us now walk down the plush, carpeted stairs together, as you slide your hand along the smooth banister. Here we go—step-ping down onto the top step—10, warm relaxed feelings spread over your entire body as your feet sink into the soft carpet. 9, feel yourself stepping down and feel the plush carpet beneath your feet. 8, you are feeling good and safe and you are some-how feeling younger and younger as you move on down, back in time, back towards when *[insert the indicated goal]*. 7, feeling more and more relaxed, feeling younger, getting younger and becoming smaller. Smaller and younger. 6 ... 5, and now a gentle darkness floats around you more and more with each step.

*Keep counting down all the way to 1. Intersperse suggestions for deep-ening relaxation and moving backwards in time. After you both get to the bottom of the staircase, say:*

And 1, at the bottom of the staircase, all the way down. Okay, BE THERE ...

## Eimer's Arm Levitation Method

This induction technique is also a rapid and relatively permissive induction technique that induces arm levitation, and can be followed by regression. This induction works very well with motivated clients but it is typically not appropriate with resistant clients. It is also a great induction to use as a lead-in to doing regression work and as a method of regressing a client.

Here is the essence of the words I (Eimer) use. The convincer is arm levitation. Trance ratification is built into the method. The regression method used is Floating Back in Time.

> *Position the client with their right or left arm (their choice) situated on an arm rest, palm resting downward and the elbow supported.*
>
> **Okay. We are going to do a hypnosis exercise in which you will experience one of your arms getting lighter and lighter and floating up all by itself into the air without your lifting it up consciously. And as that arm floats up all by itself, you will go deeper into hypnosis. So, I'd like you to begin by focusing your attention on your right [or left] arm and hand. Pick a spot on the back of your hand and focus your visual attention on that spot … Good. Keep looking at that spot and take in a few nice satisfying deep breaths … And as you inhale, notice that your hand and arm feel like they are lifting up a little bit. Each time you inhale they lift up. Notice that as you exhale, they settle down, but when you inhale, the hand and arm move up more than they move down.**
>
> **Now just breathe normally as you continue to stare at the spot on the back of your hand, and notice that the arm and hand still move up a little bit and feel a little lighter each time you inhale. Notice the physical sensations you feel in that hand, the fingers, the wrist and the forearm. As you notice the feelings in your hand, pick up the little movement sensations in the fingers … notice the twitching, the tremors, the tension, and notice how those movement sensations begin to spread throughout that hand and into the wrist … And notice those movement sensations spread up your hand and into your wrist and into your forearm with each and every breath you take and each and every word I say, regardless of the meaning of my words.**

Now to help those movement sensations spread upward so that you experience that hand and arm floating up all on their own, I'd like you to imagine that a string is tied around that wrist, and that string is connected to a great big colorful helium-filled balloon, and the balloon is your favorite color. And the balloon is light and buoyant and it is floating upward towards the ceiling ... Up, up, up towards the ceiling ... And as that balloon floats up it pulls your hand and forearm up with it. That string tugs up on your wrist and your hand and arm feel lighter and lighter. The movement sensations get bigger and bigger and that hand and arm move up, float up, more and more, as they feel lighter and lighter.

Now continue noticing the sensations in your hand and arm as you continue staring at that spot on your hand ... Your eyelids blink more frequently than before, and the more you stare the heavier those eyelids feel, and soon they will feel so heavy that they will want to close. Don't try to keep those eyelids open. Let them close so that you can feel more comfortable, and as they close you will drift and you will feel more and more relaxed and more and more absorbed ... and when those eyes finally close, you will drift down deep into hypnosis ... And that hand continues to float upward ... And you can continue to see that hand floating upward in your inner mind's eye ...

That's right! Up, up, up. Lighter and lighter. Floating upward like a balloon. And as that hand floats up, up, up, you go further and further, deeper and deeper into hypnosis ... And as you go further and further into hypnosis, and as that hand and arm float up, you float backwards in time, back in time ... And you continue to float backwards in time until you get back to X [state the age, time, place or event that you and the client have agreed for the client to go]. And as soon as that hand finds a place to stop floating, on your face or in the air, just hovering in the air, you will be back at X, and as soon as you are back at X, that hand will have found a place to stop floating. Whichever comes first is just fine. That hand can float up and land on your face, or it may

just float up to a point where it stops and hovers in the air ...
Okay. BE THERE ...

## Dabney Ewin's Rapid Eye Roll Induction

The following script is Eimer's version of Dabney Ewin's Rapid Eye Roll Induction (Ewin and Eimer, 2006). It illustrates an effective, rapid trance induction as verbalized to the patient:

Get comfortably relaxed. Close your eyes and keeping your eyelids closed just as if they are glued together, roll your eyeballs up as though you are looking at the top of your forehead, looking way, way up. Good. Keep looking up and take a deep, deep breath, the deepest breath you've ever taken and hold it. Feel it pressing against your chest as I count to three. 1 ... 2 ... 3. Now, let that breath all the way out just like a balloon collapsing, draining all the tension out of every nerve and fiber in your body. Keeping your eyelids closed, relax your eyes, and go deeper relaxed than you've ever been. Go deep down inside to find that part of you that knows you're precious, that your feelings matter, and that you own your own body, and it has to do what you tell it to do...

Pay attention only to the sound of my voice. Any other sounds you hear will be very pleasant in the background and just help you to get more comfortably relaxed. It's comforting to know that the rest of the world is going on about its business while you and I are doing ours ...

Keep your eyes relaxed, your jaws unclenched, your shoulders droopy, your arms limp and floppy, your neck and back comfortably supported by the chair ...And you can let all those muscles relax ... your abdomen soft, and with each breath you take as you exhale, just picture yourself blowing all your worries and stress, all your stress and tension, out into the atmosphere, never to return ... Your legs all loose and limp and lazy-like, and your mind as relaxed as your body. Feeling calm, safe, peaceful, and in control, comfortable, precious, and confident ...

Confident because you own your own mind, and it must think what you tell it to think. Confident because you own your own body and it must do what you tell it to do. Confident because you own your own feelings and they have to feel what you tell them to feel. Way, way, way, down deep ...

Now, I want to help you find your "Laughing Place", because laughing is healthy and drives out misery. Even if you haven't had a good laugh in a long, long time. Let your inner mind bring up a happy memory of a time when you felt like laughing and perhaps you will experience some of the feelings and sensations that go along with that memory ... the scene, the place, the colors, the shapes, the people you are with, or the quiet peacefulness of solitude, the sounds, the laughter, the music, or perhaps the voice of someone who loves you ... the smells that are here ... the touch and caresses of someone who loves you; all the things that make your laughing place, *your* laughing place, so good ... so free of any cares, or worries, or duties ... And while you are enjoying *your* laughing place, nothing can bother you and nothing can disturb you ...

When your inner mind knows that you are so concentrated on your laughing place that nothing can bother, nothing can disturb, just give me a little nod of your head so I'll know you've found it ... And having found it, take a mental snapshot of it now, so that at any time when we're doing therapy together, we can instantly shift back to this picture for comfort.

## Re-Alerting Technique #1

In a moment, I am going to alert you by counting slowly from 1 to 3. When I say 3, blink your eyes and open them, and come back fully alert, sound in mind, sound in body and in control of your feelings. 1 ... rousing up slowly ... 2 ... and 3. Wide awake, alert, refreshed, and feeling great.

*Re-Alerting Technique #2*
*An alternate alerting technique is to use a double bind by suggesting:*

> **When your deepest mind knows that you can control this symptom (or keep processing this), you'll blink your eyes and come back fully alert, sound in mind, sound in body and in control of your feelings.**

This gives the patient a choice between staying in trance forever or accepting the suggestion.

## Mental Confusion: Client Counts Backwards

I (Hunter) frequently use one of two mental confusion techniques taught by the late Charles Tebbetts. Since many professionals ask for scripts, they are included in this book. The first one involves asking the client to count backwards from 100. Say:

> **In a moment I'm going to ask you to start counting backwards from 100, only one number per breath. You may begin now with 100 ... As you count, imagine you can see or hear the numbers before you try to find them, and they're getting farther and farther away. And I'll talk to your subconscious. You don't have to try to listen, just try to find each number. And as you skip numbers, repeat numbers or forget numbers, you go deeper and deeper into hypnosis, or let go into a total trance.**

> *Listen carefully, adjusting the script whenever the client skips or repeats a number.*

> **Just relax the numbers right out of your mind, allowing them to fade farther and farther, or smaller and smaller. Forgetting to remember, or remembering to forget. It's easier and easier to forget them or just relax them away. Difficult to remember, or easy to forget. And the slightest hesitation between numbers DOUBLES your relaxation, or triples the trance ... sending you deeper into hypnosis, releasing, relaxing and letting go ... you can either forget the last number, or the next number ... or the one before that ...**

*Once your client skips a number, the critical faculty is bypassed. Continue, while interjecting words such as:*

**Very good. You're responding very good. Your conscious can either listen, or drift and wander, or both, while your subconscious is free to hear and respond to every word.**

*When your client stops counting, deepen immediately. Pay attention to your client's responses and adjust accordingly! If your client continues counting in sequence to the low eighties (or after struggling with a couple numbers), say some numbers yourself with words such as:*

**77, double the hypnosis, or triple the trance ... 75, it's so easy to imagine whatever you wish as 74 causes your conscious mind to find it so difficult even to try to look for the numbers, that on 70, it's just easier to relax and forget to count, or simply go deeper. 64, 58. Very good. Perhaps the next number was 68 ... or was it 43? It makes no difference as the count goes below 30. You just find it easier and easier to respond to my voice as you go deeper and deeper on 25. Drifting right on down. You may be surprised at how deep you go, or perhaps you'll find yourself in total trance. You may even forget to remember the numbers I speak, or you can remember to forget where you stopped counting ...**

*At this point, you may (if necessary) again enhance the mental confusion with more unrelated and incomplete sentences, or meaningless statements interjected with random numbers and suggestions for deep hypnosis.*

## Mental Confusion: Eyes Open and Close

Here is the second mental confusion technique that I (Hunter) frequently use with analytical resisters. Say:

**Find a point on the wall and stare at it. As I count backwards from 100, close your eyes on even numbers and open them on odd numbers.**

**100, just close your eyes, take a deep breath, and relax ... You may notice the mind can think many times faster than the**

spoken voice, and that's okay ... 99, open them, take another deep breath, and try to stare at that same object again ...

98, eyes closed. Very good. Just imagine you're releasing all the cares of the day as easily as you release the air from your lungs ... 97, find it's getting more difficult to even try to open your eyes. 96, eyes closed. Good. Just find yourself wanting to go deeper and deeper as you forget whether your eyes should be open or closed, or closed or open, on odd or even ...

95, easy to forget. 94, difficult to remember, whether they should be closed ... and as soon as you forget to remember, or remember to forget, or vice versa, they stay closed, and you can just relax even deeper, or let go into hypnosis. 93, good! 92 ... deeper and deeper relaxed ... It's so easy to respond to my voice as I say 91, 90 ... your eyes just want to stay closed any time now.

*Start speaking somewhat quicker and with more authority.*

88, 86. Deeper and deeper. Easy to forget, difficult to remember, 84, 82, whether they should be open or closed ... or is it closed or open ... 79, 75, 74. The numbers can skip away so quickly now that you just find yourself wanting to go deeper as your eyes want to stay closed. 72, 70. You can release yourself into deep hypnosis, or simply let go into total trance. 67, 65, 64. And every time you forget to remember, or remember to forget, open or closed, odd or even, you go deeper and deeper. 60, 50. Eyes closed and going deeper. Forgetting to remember, or remembering to forget. 40, 30. Feeling good. Responding to my voice. Releasing, relaxing, letting go. Deeper and deeper.

*Once your client leaves his/her eyes totally closed during an odd number, the moment of passivity has usually occurred. You may stop the counting if you wish and follow immediately with deepening suggestions, or continue on as part of the deepening.*

### Hunter's Variation on the Elman Rapid Induction

Although I (Hunter) rarely use rapid inductions, the one I like best is a variation on a Dave Elman induction. Sit beside your client, either on the right or the left. Place the palm of your hand (palm up) about 8 to 12 inches above the soft arm of the recliner or above the client's lap. After asking if he/she is ready to be hypnotized, say:

> As I place my palm here, place your hand, palm down, on top of mine. When you close your eyes, gradually increase the pressure as I count backwards from the number 5.
>
> Go ahead and close your eyes and take a DEEP breath ... and exhale.
>
> 5, pushing slightly on my hand. Choose hypnosis and you can go into hypnosis when I give the suggestion.
>
> 4, pushing a little harder now, breathing slowly and deeply. Let a WAVE of relaxation flow from head to toe.
>
> 3, pushing even harder now, just waiting for the suggestion to go into trance, with another WAVE of relaxation flowing from head to toe.
>
> 2.
>
> *Quickly pull your hand away and say with authority:*
>
> **DEEP TRANCE!**

Note that most clients will not be expecting the suggestion to enter hypnosis until the number 1. Giving the suggestion at number 2 adds to the element of surprise, often resulting in a deeper state of hypnosis than waiting until the last number.

# CHAPTER 4

# Phase 2: Regression Techniques to Discover the Cause

The objective of this phase is to use an appropriate regression technique to discover the cause. It is important to note that we use the word *discover* rather than diagnose.

Since there is no induction that is perfectly suitable for all of your clients all of the time, we recommend that you learn several different induction techniques at least, as well as principles for designing your own inductions that fit your client and the clinical situation. The same principle applies to hypnotic regression techniques. Regardless of the technique you learned in any previous training, we recommend that you learn a few different regression techniques in order to have choices for clients who fail to respond to the regression techniques you normally use. Additionally, we strongly recommend that the affect bridge technique (described on pages 86–90) be included in your repertoire of regression techniques. The affect bridge typically takes the client right back to either the initial sensitizing event or the activating event.

The probability of success increases with the depth of hypnosis, which is why we should take as much time as necessary to deepen our clients appropriately before beginning the second phase of a regression session. Furthermore, resistance to remembering unpleasant feelings may keep the client stuck in the present and/or result in emergence from trance; so as with the art of inducing hypnosis, it is a good idea to know more than one regression technique in order to maximize the probability of success.

It is also important to recognize that some clients remain stuck in the past, and blocked from moving forward in their lives, through the spontaneous and repeated reactivation of their uncomfortable feelings. These feelings are their connection to the past, so the *cause* of their problems can also constitute the *cure*.

Since everyone is different, it is often not obvious whether to employ regression for a particular problem. If there is any doubt about whether HRT is the right choice for your client, consider the information presented below; otherwise, move right on and choose a regression technique from those discussed in this chapter.

## The Seven Psychodynamics of a Symptom

Both authors have for years often found great clinical value in using a structured ideomotor inquiry for discovering the potential causes of their clients' presenting problems before embarking on regression therapy. The procedure is based on the "seven keys" to the psychodynamics of clients' symptoms originally presented by Cheek and LeCron in their book, *Clinical Hypnotherapy* (1968). As taught by Charles Tebbetts, and detailed in chapter 6 of Hunter's *The Art of Hypnotherapy* (2010b), we believe that most causes of emotional problems fit into one or more of these basic categories, also termed "the seven psychodynamics of a symptom."

1. **Authority imprint.** This refers to a belief that was implanted or imprinted in a client's mind by an authority figure (parent, teacher, church, government, doctor, etc.). Charles Tebbetts refers to this as "attribution" in *Miracles on Demand* (1985).

2. **Present or current unresolved issue (called "body language" by Tebbetts).** Psychosomatic illnesses (hives, migraine headaches, etc.) are often symptoms of unresolved emotional or psychological issues. This is one way that the subconscious says, "I don't like what you are doing." Charles Tebbetts called this "body language" but we prefer to call it "present or current unresolved issue," as some symptoms are undesired habits (such as overeating or smoking).

3. **Secondary gain.** The symptom sometimes offers a reward or the hope of a reward. The reward is usually insufficient to justify the suffering caused by the symptom. For example, one who is sick can get sympathy. The desire for protection or sympathy might also be the secondary gain, as with someone who stays heavy to avoid attracting someone of the opposite sex. The reward can also be punishing someone else, revenge, financial gain, attention, manipulation and so on.

4. **Identification.** This refers to identifying with a hero, mentor or loved one that someone wishes to emulate.

5. **Internal conflict.** The symptom often prevents the carrying out of a taboo desire; or there may be two conflicting desires. For example, one might stay heavy to minimize being tempted into sexual contact with others.

6. **Past experience.** This refers to the effect of a past painful event or of an event that may have been *incorrectly perceived* by the subconscious. The event may or may not be remembered accurately. Note: Not all false memories are planted by therapists! What emerges in a regression may be truth, embellishment based on facts or total fantasy believed by the subconscious. *Be certain you understand how to competently handle hypnotic regressions before attempting them.*

7. **Self-punishment.** This key refers to punishing the self because of personal guilt or to avoid possible punishment from a higher authority because of a past action, event or habit.

### Ideomotor Response Questioning for the Seven Psychodynamics

These basic questions will enable you to conduct a structured inquiry into the seven psychodynamics of a symptom, as discussed above. We consider this to be like a psychodynamic lab work-up. We ask *all seven* questions *first* before digressing into any "yes" responses provided by the client, because many clients provide a "yes" answer to more than one question. In the following section ("Evaluating Responses"), we provide guidelines for following up on "yes" responses.

First, choose your method of establishing the appropriate finger responses (as discussed in Chapter 3). Next, follow your chosen procedure immediately with the series of questions appearing below. We find most clients respond appropriately with the following wording; but if a question fails to generate a response within about 20 seconds, paraphrase with simple language. *Always keep it simple.*

**Now I'm going to ask your subconscious a series of questions related to the CAUSE of the problem ... and you may respond with "yes" or "no" or by moving the "I don't know" finger.**

1. **Is the cause related to a suggestion that was IMPRINTED in your mind by an authority figure of the past or the present?**

   ○ *Yes*  ○ *No*  ○ *I don't know, or not ready to answer yet*

2. **Is the cause related to a current UNRESOLVED ISSUE?**

   ○ *Yes*  ○ *No*  ○ *I don't know, or not ready to answer yet*

3. **Has your subconscious caused that problem because you have something else to GAIN?**

   ○ *Yes*  ○ *No*  ○ *I don't know, or not ready to answer yet*

4. **Are you IDENTIFYING with someone else?**

   ○ *Yes*  ○ *No*  ○ *I don't know, or not ready to answer yet*

5. **Are you feeling an INNER CONFLICT or two conflicting desires?**

   ○ *Yes*  ○ *No*  ○ *I don't know, or not ready to answer yet*

6. **Was your problem caused by a PAST EVENT?**

   ○ *Yes*  ○ *No*  ○ *I don't know, or not ready to answer yet*

7. **Are you PUNISHING yourself or someone else for something?**

   ○ *Yes*  ○ *No*  ○ *I don't know, or not ready to answer yet*

In some instances, you may need to consider a "don't know" response as a "yes" response. When possible, ask the subconscious to verbalize so that you may ask open-ended questions (what, when, why, where, who, how). The authors recommend that you create your own template for clients, using the above script as a guideline.

## Evaluating the Responses

Below we provide guidelines for exploring "yes" responses for each psychodynamic. Note: If the client answers "yes" to Question 2 (a current unresolved issue), this trumps all other psychodynamics; because a yes in this category may require either a referral to another professional or a conscious decision for the client to make in a fully aware state. Explore a yes response in Question 2 first before exploring any other yes responses.

Some problems have multifaceted causes, such as with overweight clients, resulting in several yes responses. Unless one of the yes responses is regarding a current unresolved issue there is no scientific protocol as to which response to explore first. We should base the decision on the combination of the client, the presenting problem and any information disclosed during previous sessions and/or the intake.

1. If "yes" to an IMPRINT from an authority figure:

   Find out which authority and any specifics about the imprint. Based on what emerges regression will probably be indicated. The treatment plan is to regress the client back to when the suggestion was made and to remove the suggestion or imprint. For example, a phobia might be an imprint passed on by a parent or grandparent.

2. If "yes" to: **Is the cause related to a current UNRESOLVED ISSUE?**

   Ask:

   > **Is your inner mind willing to allow us to use hypnotherapy to help you to resolve the problem?**

If the client signals "yes," this means that hypnotic regression therapy to the origins of the issue may be indicated. Parts therapy or one of its variations is often also indicated.

If the client signals "no" or "I don't know" to the above question, *ask the subconscious to reveal the cause of the problem to the client's conscious mind*; then re-alert the client and discuss the situation before proceeding. The unresolved issue may require psychotherapy without hypnotherapy, reality counseling or some other professional help.

3. If "yes" to: **Has your subconscious caused that problem because you have something else to GAIN?**

   Explore specifics. Is the subconscious seeking protection, attention, sympathy or leverage to manipulate someone? We may employ hypnotic regression therapy to when the subconscious first discovered that the problem could provide any of the identified secondary gains. Help the client to release attendant affect and learn a more adaptive way to get his/her needs met. Note that we could also employ parts therapy for a secondary gain.

4. If "yes" to IDENTIFYING with someone else:

   Find out who the client wants to emulate, and why. It is usually indicated to regress the client to when his/her subconscious first decided that having the problem made him or her closer to, or like, the other person. One of the authors had an overweight client years ago whose idol was an actress who gained weight for a specific part in a popular movie.

5. If "yes" to an INNER CONFLICT or two conflicting desires:

   The client needs to make a decision. Parts therapy (or one of its variations) is usually the best choice for optimal results, although HRT can often help.

6. If "yes" to a problem caused by a PAST EVENT:

   Hypnotic regression is usually the best choice.

7. If "yes" to: **Are you PUNISHING yourself or someone else for something?**

   Hypnotic regression, and/or parts therapy, and/or verbalizing are indicated. In some instances, this may require a referral for marital or family therapy (e.g., if a client is in an abusive relationship). Note that while punishing someone else is really a secondary gain, sometimes the subconscious responds with a "yes" to Question 7 rather than Question 3.

Now we will assume regression is indicated, and the preparation phase is complete.

## Regression Techniques

This section presents several different regression techniques which have been taught by some well-known hypnotherapists over the years. Remember that the goal is to discover both the initial sensitizing event and the activating event. Sometimes the ISE and AE (or symptom producing event) are combined into one event. Conversely, the subconscious occasionally requires that we discover and release one or more subsequent sensitizing events.

Some clients may respond to one regression technique for discovering the ISE on a first regression (such as the affect bridge), but may require a different technique (such as age regression) to discover the AE on a subsequent regression. Also, note that some clients will regress to the AE in the first regression, and then regress to the ISE during the second regression. Everyone is different, including two clients with a similar presenting problem; so we need to fit the technique to the client rather than vice versa.

Regardless of the technique employed, a regression becomes more powerful if relived in the present tense (revivified inside the imagination) rather than simply remembered with the logical mind, so *listen carefully* when the client responds to the "W" questions (who, what, when, where, why, how). Clients responding in the past tense are remembering rather than revivifying, which may sabotage the chances of a successful regression with lasting results.

Also, be aware of the fact that even someone who is not normally visual could become visual during an intense regression, but that does *not* mean you can now use visualization techniques in future sessions with that person. Conversely, a person who is normally visual might have difficulty describing what was seen during a childhood trauma if the sense of hearing and/or physical pain dominated their awareness at the time. Note that only some of the regression techniques detailed here incorporate imagery, although there are excellent imagery techniques for visual clients. Tad James, Ph.D., describes some valuable techniques in his book on Time Line Therapy (James & Woodsmall, 1988).

Before proceeding, remember to set aside your own preconceived opinions regarding the core cause of your client's problem(s), regardless of what the client disclosed during the pre-induction discussion or in any previous session, because over 50% of the time your opinion will be wrong (Emmerson, 2003). We mention this for the third time because of the extreme importance of avoiding inappropriate leading, and because therapists have a tendency to ignore this warning. Also note that once your client responds to the regression technique of choice, continue according to the guidelines discussed on pages 103–105.

## Affect Bridge

This technique stands out above others when strong emotions surround the client's presenting problem, and usually takes the client directly back to either the ISE or the AE.

John and Helen Watkins (1997) developed this technique decades ago. Charles Tebbetts also experimented with the same technique and called it "the feeling connection" because of the use of emotions to connect to the core cause of a problem. Roy Hunter learned this technique directly from Tebbetts in 1983 when he was one of his students; but Hunter uses the label more widely recognized in the hypnosis profession, "the affect bridge." However, the technique is based on the psychological fact that emotions, feelings or affect can activate, drive and intensify recall. Thus, feelings can bring you back to earlier times when you felt similarly.

The affect bridge technique essentially involves three steps:

1. Suggesting to the client that he/she feel an emotion or feeling linked to the presenting problem.

2. Suggesting that the feeling will intensify as you count from 1 up to 10.

3. Guiding the client back to the first time, or an earlier time, that he/she felt that same emotion as you count backwards from 10 down to 1.

The psychological principle is that feelings are a connection to the past (hence Tebbetts's use of the term)—the feeling connection. Emotions or feelings are like the glue or binding that connects the associations we make between different experiences in our memory. We often remember events based on our mood state at the time. We sort and categorize memories based on how those things make us feel—good, bad, happy, glad, mad, scared, sad, ashamed, guilty and so forth. The subconscious mind stores impressions of all of our experiences, irrespective of our ability to recall them accurately or in detail. The ease, accuracy and extent of our recall is influenced by how the original experience was registered, perceived and organized when it was first lived through and encoded in our memory.

The concept of *state dependent memory* is relevant here (Rossi & Cheek, 1994). That is, memories are often more easily retrieved and recalled when a person is in an emotional and physical state similar to the one he/she was in when the memory was first encoded. This phenomenon is commonly experienced automatically when one is listening to an old song or piece of music. You may become aware that the music makes you feel a certain way, and the feelings may bring back memories of earlier times in your life when you felt similarly; for example, when you were dating a person, had a certain job, lived in a particular place or when you were much younger.

Feelings and emotions have energy. Thus, they move you. However, they can also overwhelm and paralyze you if do not have concepts, behaviors or habits to channel the energy. As taught by Cal Banyan and others (Callahan & Trubo, 2002; Watkins, 1978), different feelings and emotions vibrate at different amplitudes and frequencies. When current situations activate particular emotions, the emotional frequencies triggered resonate with similar emotions associated with stored memories. Thus, emotions from the past can cascade into the present situation. These resonating emotions can carry old childhood behaviors and thinking into the adult present.

Emotions and feelings are our connections, or bridge, to the past. Thus, in addition to being like the glue that connects or associates one memory to another and another, feelings are also like the password that you need to access a program or data on your computer. However, you consciously type in a password, whereas you automatically have feelings. They are subconsciously driven. In doing hypnotic regression work, you, the hypnotherapist, make conscious use of this principle to guide your client back into the past, to release painful affect and change blocking beliefs that are interfering with your client's happiness.

Freud actually caught on to this principle after he rejected hypnosis as a tool for exploring his patients' unconscious minds. He developed the psychoanalytic technique of *free association* to enable patients to bring up unconscious material related to their core intrapsychic conflicts. The central principle of his psychoanalytic technique, which has remained a cornerstone of psychoanalytic psychotherapies to this day, was to ask patients who are free-associating about current complaints questions such as: "What does that remind you of?" and "Does that remind you about anything that you experienced as a child?" The keys to bringing up associations and memories are *feelings* and *emotions*— the "feeling connection" or "affect bridge."

Here is a sample script of the affect bridge technique. Add additional words as appropriate regarding the presenting problem. Also note that normal rules of grammar do not always apply with hypnotic scripts (such as using phrases rather than complete sentences).

Imagine yourself right now in a situation where [*briefly state the problem*]. As I count from 1 to 10, go deeper into the feelings you have surrounding that problem, and feel those emotions as strongly as you can. SAFELY feel them when I say 10. Number 1, go deeper into the feeling. Number 2, let the feelings grow stronger with each number. 3, stronger and stronger. 4, more powerful. 5 and 6, feeling the emotion more and more with every number you hear. 7, 8, 9, 10! Feel the feelings as strongly as you can SAFELY do so ... And now, go back to the FIRST TIME you felt those feelings as I count back to 1. 10, 9, 8, farther back in time. 7, 6, 5, way back. 4, 3, 2, back to the very first time you felt that way. 1!

BE there ... what do you see, hear or feel?

*Alternatively you may ask:*

Make a report ... what's happening?

Be very observant of the client when employing the affect bridge. If the client starts abreacting quickly, speed up your count. If the client is suppressing any evidence of emotions, count slowly and add any imagery as appropriate to associate the client into the experience. For example, here is a sample script for an analytical client with a fear of flying who tries to suppress emotions at first.

Imagine yourself right now sitting on a jet plane getting ready for takeoff. You KNOW what that feels like! Now, as I count from 1 to 10, go deeper into the feelings you have about what you are seeing, hearing and feeling; feeling those emotions as strongly and as intensely as you can, SAFELY feel them when I say the number 10.

Number 1, the plane is approaching the runway for takeoff. Notice your feelings as you sit with your seatbelt fastened, aware of the movement of the plane.

Number 2, go deeper into the feelings. Imagine looking around or out the window ... the captain says, "Flight attendants, prepare for takeoff." You feel the seat you're sitting on, sensing the movement of the plane.

Number 3, let the feelings grow stronger with each number. Imagine looking either out the window or around the cabin.

Number 4 ... stronger and stronger. Hear the sound of the jet engines revving up for takeoff. Imagine looking around if you wish.

Number 5. Feel the plane accelerating, hear the sound of the jet engines and feel yourself being pressed into the seat.

Number 6, feel the emotion more and more with every number you hear, and the plane climbs into the air.

Number 7, hear or feel the plane vibrating as it climbs higher and higher, pressing you farther back in your seat ... or look out the window or at the other passengers as you go into those feelings.

Number 8, higher and higher, stronger and stronger.

Number 9, you KNOW what it feels like to fly ... BE there in your mind!

10! Feel the feelings as strongly as you can SAFELY do so ... and now go back to the FIRST TIME you felt those feelings as I count back to 1. 10, 9, 8, farther back. 7, 6, 5, way back. 4, 3, 2, back to the very first time you felt that way. 1! BE THERE ... what do you see, hear or feel?

Note that you can shorten the above script as the client displays any sign of emotional discomfort. Also, once the client responds to your first question above, continue according to the guidelines discussed on pages 103–105. If the client fails to respond, choose a different regression technique.

An alternative technique to the affect bridge is the "time tunneling technique." I (Eimer) learned this technique from Cal Banyan during one of his 5-PATH® intensive trainings. The essence of the verbalization as I say it is as follows:

**Would you like to be free of that feeling of** *[insert what the client calls the feeling]* **forever?**

*Wait for an answer:*

**Okay. Good. Get into the feeling then. You are safe here in my office. Focus on that feeling of ... You can describe the feeling to me if you wish. Make that feeling as real and as powerful as it's ever been.**

**Now, imagine that this feeling is a tunnel ... A tunnel into the past. A tunnel that goes all the way back to the very first time you felt that way ... Now, mentally go into that tunnel, surrounded by that feeling in your body. And mentally go back through that tunnel into the past ... to when that feeling starts. Follow it back. It's connected to every time in your life you felt that way. Notice the end of the tunnel. Follow the tunnel to its end and raise this index finger** *[stroke client's index finger]* **when you come out at the end of the tunnel.**

*Wait for the finger signal. Then say:*

**Good. Now that you have come to the end of the tunnel, tell me your first impressions. What's happening?**

*Further inquiry:*

**Are you inside or outside? Are you alone or with other people? Is it daytime or nighttime? What are you doing? How old are you? What are you feeling? What are you thinking?**

Before using the affect tunnel technique, verify that your client is comfortable with the imagery of a tunnel.

## Age Regression

The affect bridge and affect tunnel techniques are essentially *symptom regressions* as we guide the client back in time using the symptom or feeling as a bridge or tunnel into the past to earlier times, or the first time that the client felt the symptom or feeling. Many people consider age regression to apply to any hypnotic regression to a time in our current life, regardless of the regression technique employed; however, the term "age regression" also refers to an actual regression technique. It is easy to understand why so many people share the above opinion, because *age regression* is the most widely used regression technique.

There are two primary age regression methods: counting backwards by age, or counting forwards from zero (representing infancy). Most hypnotherapists using age regression count backwards. Hollywood has used this technique in several movies; nonetheless, it can be effective with many people when properly employed. After deepening to at least a medium level of trance, say words such as:

> **Now take a deep breath and go deeper and deeper into a deep, pleasant, hypnotic sleep …**
>
> *Speak very slowly and softly. Take a long, deep breath before each sentence and "sigh" the words as though you were sleepy.*
>
> **Now you are drifting back in time. Just imagine you're going back in time to when you were 40 …** *[provided client is over 40!]* **Going back to a VERY important event … 35 … further back … 30 … Let the years fade away … 25 … 20 … Please answer with your fingers, "yes" or "no." Did the important event happen before age 20?**
>
> *If the "no" or "I don't know" finger moves, ask the client to stop you when you get to a very important age, and count forward from 20. If the "yes" finger moves (more common), continue:*
>
> **Please stop me or move the "yes" finger when we get to a very important age when a VERY important event happens. 19 … 18 … 17 … 16 … 15 …**
>
> **Stop me when we get to a very important year … 14 … 13 … 12 … Stop me when something very relevant to that problem happens … 11 … 10 … You feel your body getting smaller … 9 … Your arms and legs becoming shorter … 8 … going back to a very important age … 7 … 6 … 5 … very small now … 4 … even younger … something important happens … BE THERE!**

*Whenever the client stops you and speaks, listen and proceed accordingly. If he/she displays any emotions or abreactions, or moves the "yes" or "I don't know" finger, stop the script and say:*

**Make a report. WHAT'S HAPPENING?**

*If the client does not stop you after you get to number 4, continue:*

**Now you are 4 and getting even smaller ... 3 ... a very early age ... 2. You are a toddler ... 1 ... something very important happens ... tell me about it ...**

**INFANCY ... Something very important happens ... BE THERE! What's happening?**

*If there is no answer, tap gently on the client's forehead or the back of the hand (you must have already obtained permission to touch) and say with more authority:*

**Answer quickly now—the first thing that comes to your mind— inside or outside?**

*As soon as client answers, continue with:*

**Are you alone or with others?**

*Wait for a response. The client may start describing details at this point. If so, listen to the dialogue and deal with what emerges. If the response is "with others," ask who; but if the response is simply the word "alone," continue with:*

**What do you see, hear or feel?**

Charles Tebbetts taught that even if the client answers one of these last three questions just to satisfy the suggestion, it is most likely the correct start for uncovering the repressed material. He believed that this line of questioning leads to a report that makes it more apparent which questions to ask next as the story unfolds. Our experience validates what Tebbetts taught.

Occasionally a client fails to stop the facilitator on any number, all the way to zero; and fails to respond to the above questions. When that happens, we can either count *forwards* from zero or use another regression technique.

Here is the rarely used age regression counting forwards:

> **Now take a deep breath and go deeper and deeper into a deep, pleasant, hypnotic sleep ...**
>
> *Speak very slowly and softly. Take a long, deep breath before each sentence and "sigh" the words as though you were sleepy. Watch the client for any evidence of abreactions as you count.*
>
> **You are drifting back in time ... going back all the way to your teens, and earlier ... through childhood, back to when you were a toddler or an infant. The problem may have started either during infancy or during any age after infancy. As I start counting, please STOP me by speaking or moving the "yes" finger when I get to a very important age. Zero represents infancy.**
>
> **Zero ... infancy...**
>
> **1 ... you are a toddler.**
>
> **2 ... you are walking now.**
>
> **3 ... you are starting to talk.**
>
> **4 ... getting bigger now.**
>
> **5 ... stop me when I get to a very important age.**
>
> **6 ... still growing.**
>
> **7 ... school age.**
>
> **8 ... stop me when something very important happens.**
>
> **9 ... your subconscious knows when to stop me.**
>
> **10 ... growing more.**
>
> **11 ... getting bigger now.**
>
> **12 ... almost in your teens.**

**13 ... you are a teenager now.**

**14 ... growing up.**

**15 ... your subconscious knows when to stop me.**

**16 ... old enough for high school.**

**17 ... growing up more now.**

**18 ... you are a legal adult.**

**19 ... please answer with your fingers, yes or no. Did the important event happen before age 20?**

*If either the "yes" or "I don't know" finger moves, count backwards from 19, asking for a finger response at each age. If the "no" finger moves, continue counting forwards from 20 until the client stops you, making certain not to count higher than the client's current age. If the client fails to respond, use another regression technique.*

Some hypnotherapists count forwards as their first choice for age regression rather than counting backwards. There is no right or wrong choice, as either method might work, or both may fail with some clients. If the client responds, continue according to the guidelines discussed on pages 103–105. If the client fails to respond to age regression, choose another regression technique.

### Regression by Calendar Years

This technique is very similar to age regression, except that the count is by calendar year rather than by the age. After deepening to at least a medium level of trance, say words such as:

**Now as you take a deep breath and go deeper and deeper into a deep, pleasant, hypnotic sleep ...**

*Speak very slowly and softly. Take a long, deep breath before each sentence and "sigh" the words as though you were sleepy.*

You are drifting back in time. Just imagine you are going back in time to *[choose a year either five or ten years ago, depending on the client's age and information known about the presenting problem]*.

Answer with your fingers, yes or no. Did the very important event happen BEFORE that year?

*If "no" or "I don't know," ask:* Did the very important event happen during that year? *[state year] If "no" or "I don't know" to that year, ask:* Did the very important event happen during the next year? *State the next year and continue asking the same question for each successive year progressing forward until you get a "yes" response.*

*If the client answers "yes," that the very important event did happen BEFORE the year you mentioned first, then continue backwards in the manner described, starting with the year preceding the first one used. For example, if the first year used was 2007, continue as follows:*

As I continue mentioning the year, stop me when I get to a VERY important year ... 2006. Either move the "yes" finger or stop me when I mention the year that reminds you of a VERY important event ... 2005.

Now the year is 2004 ... 2003 ... 2002 ... going back farther in time.

2001 ... 2000 ... 1999 ... 1998 ... Stop me when I get to a very important year.

Going back ... 1997 ... Farther back. Let the years roll backward, going back in time ... 1996 ... Stop me when we get to a very important year ...

*And so on. We may count the first few years by fives if the client is over 40.*

It is important to know the date of the client's birth if using regression by calendar years in order to avoid counting back before the client's birth. If the client responds, continue according to the guidelines discussed on pages 103–105. If the client fails to respond, choose another regression technique.

## Pleasant Time and Place

If the client fails to regress by age or calendar years, we may consider another technique that Charles Tebbetts taught in his classroom. Simply suggest going back to a very happy time out of childhood. This can be an enjoyable birthday party, a wonderful holiday or vacation experience and so forth. Once there, we may simply ask the client to describe what is happening or what can be seen, heard and felt. Then we may move either forward or backward to a very relevant event.

As both authors have discovered from experience, this technique might not be effective with clients who experienced a very sad childhood; so you may wish to consider an imagery technique instead.

## Hallway of Time

Using the imaginary hallway of time can be quite effective for clients who can visualize. However, this technique can also be adapted for primarily auditory or kinesthetic clients. It involves imagery of the client opening a door into a long hallway with doors on both sides. Each door has a number corresponding to the age of the client, beginning at zero. You may edit and adapt the following script based on whether or not the client visualizes.

> Imagine that you are opening the door to a long hallway, the hallway of time. Walk through the door, and either feel yourself close it, or hear it closing behind you.
>
> There are many doorways in front of you, with numbers representing your age. Odd numbered doors are on the left, with even numbered doors on the right, starting with zero. You can see the numbers on each door, or hear the number spoken as you walk by each door.
>
> Your subconscious, your inner mind, knows which door you need to enter, and can guide you to the correct door. Permit your subconscious or inner mind to guide you to the correct door. Feel yourself drawn to the doorway to the cause of that problem. The door will either open for you, or you will find yourself reaching for the doorknob of the correct door. That door opens to another time and place, to a very important event.

> **When the door opens for you, or you open the correct door, move through it. Then raise your "yes" finger and tell me where you are …**
>
> *When the client moves either the "yes" or "I don't know" finger, ask:*
>
> **Be there … what do you see, hear or feel?**
>
> *Or ask:*
>
> **Make a report … what's happening?**

If the client responds, continue according to the guidelines discussed on pages 103–105. If the client fails to respond, choose another regression technique. Note that you may edit the above script according to the needs of the client.

## Specific Event

Sometimes a client might need to remember a specific event from the more recent past, such as a store owner who told her hypnotherapist that she could not remember where she put her deposit of the daily receipts. (She had seen a shady character loitering in her store, and hid the money so well that not even she could find it!) During the pre-induction interview, she described when she last remembered having the envelope. After appropriate deepening, she was regressed to the very same place of her last conscious memory, and asked to relive everything in her imagination just as it was happening. To her surprise, hypnosis helped her remember exactly where she decided to stash the cash. A subsequent phone call from the excited client confirmed that she had found her money. The protocol for using hypnotic regression for helping a client find a lost object is:

1.  Confirm the purpose of the session.

2.  Conduct your intake during which you have the client describe when he/she last remembered having possession of the object.

3.  Give a pre-hypnosis talk to explain what hypnosis and regression are and what they are not.

4.  Induce hypnosis and deepen the client to an appropriate level.

5.  After appropriate deepening, regress the client to his/her last conscious memory of having the object, and ask the client to relive everything in his/her imagination just as it was happening. Here we are not as worried about leading questions as we would be in HRT. We question the client to direct his/her attention to areas that might lead to striking "pay dirt."

6.  We proceed with an appropriate amount of exploration before emerging the client from hypnosis. This hopefully is when the client arrives at a point where he/she experiences him/herself putting the object in a verifiable place.

7.  Before the client is emerged, the re-alerting suggestion is given that "Your eyes will open and you will emerge from hypnosis alert and awake when your subconscious mind knows that you have uncovered all of the available information you can uncover and need to uncover at this point."

8.  After emerging the client from trance, the material relived in trance is consciously discussed and processed.

9.  Telephone follow-up is conducted within an agreed upon time to check results.

If the specific event involves a forensic application of hypnosis (such as witnessing a crime or being a victim of a crime), remember to seek proper training before venturing into that area. There are very specific legal and ethical guidelines for conducting forensic and investigative hypnosis (Eimer & Gravitz, 2007; Hammond et al., 1995; Wester & Hammond, 2011). In most states, hypnotically refreshed testimony is not admissible in court unless very specific guidelines are followed in the conducting of the forensic hypnosis sessions. In fact, in some states, hypnosis is not admissible in court at all, and can disqualify a hypnotized witness from testifying. However, in many applications of forensic hypnosis, hypnosis is used way before court, in order to obtain leads in investigations that have become cold. Nevertheless, even then, the hypnotist must have the appropriate training, must comply with all laws of the jurisdiction in which the investigation is being conducted and must avoid leading the subject.

Hypnotic regression techniques play a major role in the forensic and investigative uses of hypnosis. That is because in these applications, the goal is to use hypnosis to refresh a client's memory of past events. The techniques employed typically take the client back (regress) to the incidents in question in order to elicit information that can shed more light on the investigation. However, while the search is for the truth (i.e., the facts of the case) in forensics, we know that all memory is a reconstruction, and hence subject to distortions, whether or not the memories are hypnotically refreshed. Hence, in a forensic context, all information about past events elicited through hypnosis must be independently corroborated. In the forensic hypnosis application of regression techniques, we must be especially careful not to ask any leading questions.

Any hypnosis professional interested in forensic applications of hypnosis is advised to visit the website of one of the foremost authorities on forensic hypnosis, Marx Howell (www.marxhowell.com) (see also Brown, Hammond & Scheflin, 1998; Hammond et al., 1995).

Returning to the clinical context, sometimes a client will insist on regression back to a specific event that he/she believes is the cause of a problem. Charles Tebbetts wrote the following advice in *Miracles on Demand*:

> If you have gained relevant information in your pre-induction interview, you may regress the client to a certain date and time. You may even allow her to relive her birth experience if birth trauma is a suspected cause of the problem. (1985: 23)

Over two years before the writing of this book, Roy Hunter had a client who insisted that his fear of elevators started with a specific event involving a fire. After clearing the event discussed in the intake, it turned out to be the AE; and the ISE needed to be discovered and released in a subsequent session in order for the client to enjoy lasting success.

Another client Roy saw years ago was a hypnotherapist who insisted that his confidence problem started during a severe punishment at age five. The client believed that it was the ISE for his problem; and since Roy considers the client to be his employer, he honored the request. As it turned out, there were no abreactions because that event had already been cleared months earlier by another hypnotherapist facilitating HRT. Furthermore, his subconscious indicated that the specific childhood event had no connection to his confidence problem. Instead, the ISE for this particular problem occurred during his early twenties when a business partner broke trust and caused the client a financial disaster. Nonetheless, the client retained his belief that the childhood event may still have been connected to the loss involving his former partner. What is important is that trance persistence paid off for this man.

If you follow a client's request to regress to a specific event, be certain to ask the subconscious whether there is anything else to discover and release before concluding the session. Keep an open mind and recognize that a client's conscious belief about when and where a problem originated is usually just the tip of the iceberg. For clinical problems, regression to a specific event seldom brings up *the real core cause* of the client's problem, and further regressions and/or progressions are usually necessary. Solving the presenting problem through regression to a specific event is typically limited to helping clients remember where they put lost items, as illustrated in the cases above. Even in forensic applications of hypnosis, with very few exceptions, multiple regressions are typically necessary.

### Deck of Time
After the client or patient is in trance, say words such as the following:

> I'd like you to imagine a very special deck of cards using all of your senses. This is a very special deck of cards because instead of the familiar numbers and suits that you usually see on a usual deck of cards, in this deck, each card has a photograph of an important memory, of an important time or event in your life. In this deck, each card displays a picture of an important

scene from your life. Please imagine that you are holding this deck of cards ... feel the deck, feel the texture, smell the cards, feel the edges of the cards, and so on. Now, notice the picture on the top card in the deck.

In a moment, but not yet, I am going to ask you to shuffle the cards. When you shuffle the cards, notice what it feels like to shuffle the cards. And after you finish shuffling the cards, you will put the deck face down and then pick up the top card. When you turn up the first card, there will be a picture of *[the event, age or earlier experience of symptom or problem you are regressing the patient back to]*. You will look at that picture and let that picture take you back in time to what is happening in that picture ... so that then you will be there in the picture ...

Okay. Now shuffle the cards and when you have finished shuffling the cards, put the deck face down, pick up the top card, turn it over and look at the picture on that card. It will be a picture of X. Let that picture take you back in time into what is happening in the picture ... And be there.

*If you want the patient to go further back:*

Now just pull up one of the cards farther back in the deck, and look at the picture on that card. It will be a scene of X.

Continue according to the guidelines discussed on pages 103–105.

## Other Imagery Techniques

An occasional client might resist several regression techniques. Although Time Line Therapy promoted by Tad James is quite popular (James & Woodsmall, 1988), sometimes Roy Hunter simply asks the client the following question:

I would like to ask your subconscious or your inner mind a question: What is the best way to guide you back to the event that must be discovered?

One client told Roy to have him imagine *going down a long slide into the past*. Another said to have her enter an *elevator through time* starting at the fiftieth floor (representing her current age) of a skyscraper, and going down to the floor representing the age when the important event occurred.

Although both clients in these examples experienced successful regressions, the risk of using either technique with most clients is as follows: (1) a client with a fear of heights would reject the slide, and (2) anyone with claustrophobia (or fear of elevators) would reject the elevator through time. If you use any imagery technique other than the hallway of time, it is wise to confirm its acceptability with the client in advance, unless the client supplied the imagery as in the above two examples.

Note that the number of regression techniques might be as limitless as the imagination. We have only covered the more common ones in this book. If you obtain successful results with an effective technique not mentioned here, continue using it. However, for the benefit of your clients, master several additional regression techniques in order to help a client who fails to respond to your normal technique of choice. In addition, master the affect bridge technique. The authors have employed every regression technique discussed in this chapter at one time or another.

Once the client responds to a regression technique, continue according to the guidelines discussed in the next section.

## Facilitating the Regression

When the client starts responding, it is important that we tune our listening skills. In addition, ask open-ended questions (who, what, where, when, why, how). Common starting questions were presented in some of the regression scripts earlier in this chapter, such as:

> **What do you see, hear or feel?**

After the initial response, a good question to ask is:

| **What happens next?**

There is no script available at this point, because we should base the next question on information disclosed by the client. For example, if the client says someone is hitting him, ask *who*. If a client says, "Daddy is punishing me," then ask either *why* or *how* he is punishing, or both questions.

If the client starts displaying emotions, move on to Phase 3, covered in the next chapter. However, an analytical client will often test our listening skills; so we will discuss some important information before moving into Phase 3.

Pay very close attention to whether the client is speaking in *the present tense*, as if experiencing it in the imagination (revivifying), or speaking in the *past tense* as if simply remembering. Once a client gets to the relevant event, we must do our best to help the client relive the event as though it is currently happening in the imagination all over again. Why? This is because it is much easier to help clear the emotion if the event is re-enacted (or revivified) *in the imagination* rather than simply remembered with the conscious mind. Analytical clients tend to remember as a form of analytical resistance, stuffing the emotions back into the subconscious.

## Keeping Your Client in the Regression

When a client starts suppressing emotions by speaking in the past tense, ask:

| **Imagine you are there again ... what's happening NOW, and how does that make you feel?**

If the client stays in a "left brain" mode of remembering, he/she may even bounce out of hypnosis if we do not respond quickly. If this starts to happen, then simply suggest:

> **Experience it in your imagination as though it is happening NOW. Feel the experience and make a report.**

Sometimes a client might still resist responding in the present tense, in which case it may be necessary to employ further deepening techniques. In such a case, it is acceptable to use regression back to the specific event described, provided the client gave enough information; otherwise, it may be necessary to use another regression technique.

In a regression therapy session some years ago, one of Roy's clients kept remembering rather than regressing even after two different regression techniques—and then opened her eyes and said, "It's not working!" Roy reminded her to go into her feelings and relive the scene in her imagination, then asked her to close her eyes. After a couple more deepening techniques, the affect bridge technique (which she originally resisted) finally got her totally into a past emotional event, resulting in a successful outcome.

### When to Move On ...

Once we have discovered the cause, we have accomplished the second of the four primary hypnotherapy objectives discussed in Chapter 1 of this book; but we must use the guidelines discussed in this section until the client displays some sort of emotion surrounding the event. However, let us now assume our textbook client is finally in a regression back to the core cause of a problem and responding appropriately. Once the client displays abreactions, that is the bridge into the next phase of HRT, *abreactions and release*, covered in the next chapter.

# CHAPTER 5

# Phase 3: Abreactions and Release

Emotional discharges during a hypnotic regression are called *abreactions*. When the client starts displaying any abreactions, no matter how mild, that is the start of the third phase of hypnotic regression therapy.

Some hypnotherapists are afraid of abreactions and unwisely jerk a client up out of hypnosis; but doing so leaves a client stuck with the problem. Worse yet, the emotions surrounding a problem may remain at a conscious level, causing the client to pay more attention to the problem rather than the resolution. Sadly, as of the writing of this book, there are some hypnosis instructors who actually teach their students to re-alert a client immediately if abreactions occur. The authors believe this is unwise.

Other hypnotherapists use dissociation by asking the client either to become a third party observer to the event or to imagine viewing the event on a movie screen. While the argument for this approach is that it is more gentle for the client, and does not re-traumatize them, many clients need to *feel* the emotion in order to completely release it. One of the authors has experienced two unsuccessful regressions at different times because one of the two dissociative hypnotic regression techniques mentioned above was employed in order to avoid dealing with abreactions.

Conversely, a handful of hypnotherapists use very confrontational imagery during abreactions, such as asking the client to pound a pillow as though he/she is hitting the real or imagined perpetrator of the cause. One of the authors observed Gil Boyne facilitating a regression in the 1980s, asking a stutterer to pound a pillow. Even though Boyne was very paternal and authoritarian, the client enjoyed lasting success. Randal Churchill, originally trained by Boyne, also uses a confrontive style. Churchill has probably facilitated more regressions than almost anyone alive, and he obtains excellent results, as evidenced by his sessions described in his regression books (Churchill, 2002, 2008).

Charles Tebbetts, who also learned regression techniques from Boyne, used a less confrontive style that is more client centered. The authors believe that the client centered approach is more considerate of clients. In other words, neither force nor inhibit abreactions, but *allow* clients to discharge emotions *in their own ways*. That being said, using either dissociation or a paternal approach is not incorrect when the client obtains successful results.

We should also avoid interfering during abreactions. This is *not* the time to offer advice or share our experiences. Rather, it is of utmost importance to be a good listener, regardless of whether the client cries or swears, and so on.

## Types of Abreactions

There are three main types of abreactions: intense, moderate or minimal; and some clients will suppress the abreactions. We should consider handling each of these types of abreactions differently in order to facilitate them in a client centered manner. Note that some clients will try to suppress emotional discharges even though speaking in the present tense. In any event, have a box of tissues nearby, as even middle-aged men sometimes cry profusely during hypnotic regression therapy.

### Intense Abreactions

Some people are so close to their feelings that they may actually experience abreactions outside of a formal hypnotic trance simply by talking about a past event. For this reason, psychotherapists and mental health counselors who have clients talk about the past may wish to consider formal training in hypnotherapy and HRT so that they can spot the spontaneous trance, or at least obtain training in regression therapy in order to avoid inappropriate leading.

When a regressed client starts an intense abreaction (such as sobbing, screaming, loud swearing, etc.), we may use one of the two options described below if we need to reduce the emotional intensity of the abreaction. In addition, place a tissue in the client's hand.

1. *Emotional distancing (or dissociation):*

   **Now you can imagine either that you are observing the event as an invisible observer, or imagine that you are watching it on a movie screen. Please tell me which is easier for you ...**

   *Use the imagery the client chooses. Then ask the "W" questions, listen and deal with what emerges.*

2. *Reduction of intensity:*

   **Let the scene fade away now and go back to your safe and peaceful place, or a scene in which you are HAPPY and enjoying yourself thoroughly. Be there, feeling how wonderful life is at this moment in time ... or simply go back to your safe and peaceful place. Take a deep breath and RELAX, and just feel how wonderful life is at this moment.**

   **It is important to your future happiness that you go back to the previous scene you just experienced—but this time the feelings will be much less intense. For the sake of your happiness, are you willing to go back to that scene for just a short moment?**

   *After obtaining a "yes" response, proceed appropriately with "W" questions, competently dealing with what emerges.*

While most clients do not need either of the above techniques, the client centered approach is to use dissociation with the person who feels very intense emotions during a regression.

## Moderate Abreactions

Clients displaying moderate abreactions are the most common, and fortunately the easiest to help. There may be some crying (though not intense) and/or tears with some feelings verbalized, in which case we may still place a tissue in the client's hand.

Simply allow the client to abreact, and be a good listener. Once the initial abreactions start subsiding, we can move on to the next step as discussed in the next major section.

## Minimal Abreactions

Close observation of the client's facial expressions and non-verbal language (e.g., tone of voice) can help the hypnotherapist determine whether the client is feeling any emotion. Sometimes the evidence might be one lone tear, the trembling of a hand or a few swear words.

We can still proceed to ask the "W" questions until enough information is gathered to identify a core cause that can be released. Listen carefully to be sure that the client is not suppressing the emotions accompanying the event.

## Suppressed Abreactions

A handful of clients attempt to suppress or avoid abreactions altogether even though talking in the present tense. When this happens, we can *invite* the abreaction by asking:

> **How does that make you FEEL?**

Emphasize the word "feel." The above question has worked well for both of the authors over the years, as hypnotherapists and as clients. After asking the question, listen carefully to the response. If the client starts verbalizing feelings, proceed with more "W" questions as appropriate. If the client makes further attempts to suppress emotions by either talking in the past tense or by saying something like "I think he should be nicer to me," and so on, then use a phrase such as the following:

> **Do not try to think about it. Instead, tell me exactly how that makes you FEEL ...**

Note the use of the word "try" in the above statement, combined with "do not." The subconscious ignores the negative (e.g., "Don't think of a dog"), while the conscious mind hears the whole statement. Meanwhile, the word "try" implies failure to the subconscious; and we do *not* want the client to think about the process. Instead, he/she needs to *feel* the experience in order to more easily release it and have a successful catharsis. Roy has used the above two sentences with analytical clients successfully over a period of many years.

## Peaceful Place and Informed Child Technique

When the abreactions start to subside and we have enough information disclosed regarding the event discovered by the regression technique, we may now guide the client back to his/her peaceful (or safe) place. There is no scientific point at which we can say dogmatically that it is time to do so; rather, that decision is often made intuitively based on being a good listener and observer. While it is not a serious problem if we keep the client in the regression too long, doing so can sometimes provide a little more emotional discomfort than necessary for facilitating release. However, taking the client out of the event too soon might inhibit a complete release. So use good clinical judgment to titrate it just right for that particular client.

When appropriate, say:

> Now go to your peaceful place. Take a deep breath, and RELAX …

If appropriate, you may give the client a few more suggestions to deepen the hypnotic state and/or rest for a minute or so before employing the informed child technique. When ready, say:

> In a moment, I'm going to ask you to go back to that same event, but with ALL of your present adult wisdom, knowledge, understanding, training and experience.
>
> Now … go back to that event once again and BE the *[age at regression]*-year-old, but with your present adult awareness.

111

> You just *[summarize event]* ... **What is your NEW perception of that event?**

Listen carefully, and then facilitate Gestalt role play.

## Gestalt Role Play

Fritz Perls is recognized as a pioneer of Gestalt therapy, which many psychotherapists and psychologists have used over the decades. Gil Boyne employed and taught regression therapy with the use of Gestalt role play as an important step of the releasing process (Boyne, 1989). Randal Churchill also combines Gestalt with his hypnotic regressions (Churchill, 2002). David Quigley, a former student of Churchill, does so as well (Quigley, 2011).

When I (Hunter) studied hypnosis in 1983, Charles Tebbetts showed an old video of Perls facilitating Gestalt role play with several clients. Tebbetts taught that the combination of hypnosis and regression therapy greatly enhanced the effectiveness of Gestalt therapy; and he personally told me that a regression without Gestalt would make it much more difficult for the client to obtain total release from the problem. Note that he also gave credit to Gil Boyne for teaching him how to combine Gestalt with regression.

Additionally, Tebbetts taught that Gestalt role play helps the client establish understanding at a subconscious level, which is often a prerequisite to release (Tebbetts, 1985). Whether or not someone agrees with that opinion, tens of thousands of client successes have resulted from sessions facilitated by the practitioners mentioned above.

### What to Say and Do
After the client tells you his/her new perception of the event, ask the client to speak to the real or imagined perpetrator first. If more than one person is involved (such as a sibling and a parent), let the client choose which person to speak to first, and *where* to speak to that person. Make it safe for the client to talk by saying words such as:

> **Imagine that** *[name of other person]* **is in front of you right now.**
> **He** *[or she]* **MUST LISTEN to everything you have to say. Tell**
> **that person exactly how his [or her] actions hurt you then, and**
> **in the years that followed. Say,** *[name]* **you made me feel ...**
>
> *Listen carefully. If client fails to start talking within about 30 seconds,*
> *paraphrase the above and again ask the client to speak. Remind the cli-*
> *ent that it is now SAFE to speak to that person.*
>
> **He [or she] must now listen to you talk. Remember, you have all**
> **your present adult knowledge, wisdom, understanding, intel-**
> **ligence and experience. Tell her** *[him or them]* **EXACTLY how you**
> **FEEL about what has happened, and how it affected you then**
> **and in the years that followed ...**
>
> *Wait for response, and allow the client to speak and express his/her*
> *feelings. He/she may talk for several minutes.*

Avoid interrupting, but if you accidently do so, quickly apologize and ask the client to please continue. After listening until the client finishes, ask the client if he/she has anything more to add—and listen again. When the client has fully vented, it is time to change roles. Say:

> **Now, BE YOUR MOTHER** *[or father, or the person or animal who*
> *caused the hurt]* **and RESPOND!**

If there is no immediate response, you may repeat the phrase and then summarize what the client expressed as though you are talking to that person rather than the client:

> **Now, BE YOUR MOTHER** *[or father, or the person or animal who*
> *caused the hurt]* **... Your son** *[or daughter, brother, etc.]* **says that you**
> *[summarize whatever was done].* **He** *[or she]* **doesn't know how you**
> **can love her and do that! RESPOND TO** *[client name]***!**

Note that we must remain objective and avoid siding with either role taken during the role play (Churchill, 2002). Listen to each role carefully, eventually asking the client if he/she has anything else they wish to say to the other person. Go back and forth several times, and then ask:

> **Do you now release** [name or title of perpetrator] **from the apology they used to owe you?**

Then, last but not least, ask:

> **Are you now willing to forgive yourself and release yourself from carrying all that hurt for all these years?**

If more than one person was involved in the event, ask the client whether he/she wishes to talk to the other person(s) involved. If so, then repeat the above process. Occasionally a client resists releasing a perpetrator, as discussed in the next section.

### Helping the Resistant Client

An occasional client might say that he/she can *never* forgive that person for what was done. However, even when the client knows that the other person is still living and unwilling to change, he/she can still "give the problem back" to the other person to deal with at another time and place. If forgiveness of the perpetrator is not an option for the client, then at least seek to help the client obtain a greater understanding and expanded perspective, as this is often essential to release.

> **Do you now release** [name or title of perpetrator] **to his/her Higher Power or karma; and without condoning, do you give him/her the problem back to deal with it at another time and place?**

The above question often helps when the client is convinced that the perpetrator will not change. One of the authors helped a woman over 20 years ago who had claustrophobia. The cause was a sibling who locked her in the closet frequently when their mother was at work. While playing the role of the sadistic sister, it became evident that the sister could never feel remorse; but the above question resulted in successful release. The following week she rode up and down an elevator several times comfortably for the first time in her life.

On rare occasions, a client is still unable to release, even when the above question is asked. If that happens, then simply ask:

**What would it take for you to release** *[name or title of perpetrator]*?

Several years ago, a man was upset that his father (still living) continued to tell him how to live his life. His response to the above question was: "Take me to my safe place, where I can take the sword of truth and cut the black cords that Dad tied around me; and then ask me to surround myself with light to prevent him from attaching any more cords to me." The guided imagery proved successful for that client.

A third form of resistance may result from guilt and/or self-punishment, as sometimes a client is unable or unwilling to forgive him/herself. If this happens, ask:

**What would it take for you to forgive or release yourself?** *[And/ or]* **Haven't you suffered enough?**

Deal with what emerges, and act accordingly. Do *not* take it upon yourself to supply imagery for release, as the client might strongly dislike your chosen imagery technique. I (Hunter) made a very unwise and costly statement in 1985 with a Jewish woman after mistakenly assuming she was a Christian. After telling her to release the problem into the light of Christ, she immediately broke trance saying, "I'm Jewish, and I resent your using the name of Christ in this session!" She verbally accepted my apology, but never returned for a follow-up session.

Be sure to keep your questions open ended, without engaging in inappropriate leading. If the therapist projects his/her agenda of spiritual or professional beliefs onto the client, the session may backfire and go "south" rapidly, without any lasting results. Let the client's subconscious tell you how to complete the release.

## Confirming Release

Even after successful employment of Gestalt therapy, we cannot assume the job is complete. Instead, we should guide the client back to his/her peaceful (or safe) place and confirm release with ideomotor response signals. We should first confirm release of the particular event, and then confirm release of the problem and its causes, in that order. The reason for confirming release of the event first is that we often do not yet know whether the client needs to do Gestalt with another participant in the significant event before being able to release the problem and its causes.

### Is the Event Released?

We can confirm release of the event with a question such as:

> **Please answer with the appropriate finger response. Is that EVENT successfully released?**

The reason for the ideomotor response is that an occasional client answers a verbal "yes" while moving either the "no" or "I don't know" finger, in which case we should accept the ideomotor response.

When clients fail to confirm release of the event, it is usually because there is another perpetrator (person or animal) involved in the incident that must be forgiven or released; and we need to ask the client whom else he/she needs to talk to. One of the authors had a client in 2010 who needed Gestalt role play with a parent who was *not* present during a fight with a sibling. In another case, a client in Gestalt therapy talked to a teacher who should have supervised recess at school when he was bullied.

If the client does not provide a clear answer when you ask who else they wish to talk to, but still seem reluctant to release the event, then ask:

> **What will it take for you to completely release that event?**

Deal with what emerges. One of the authors had a client who responded to the above question by saying she wanted to give her burden to an angel. Release occurred with object projection (i.e., giving the problem a shape, color and size and projecting it outside herself). This was combined with imagery of a sacred place where she could then imagine giving the object to an angel. Another client said that she needed to bury her problem in the ground, fertilize it and let it grow into a lotus. After she moved forward in time in her mind to observe the growing lotus, release was confirmed.

If you are running out of time, it is acceptable to pause the regression at this point and continue in a subsequent session, even if the client wishes to do Gestalt role play with another perpetrator. However, it is the opinion of the authors that interrupting the session earlier than the release of at least one perpetrator from an event is not considerate of the client, and should only be done if the session must be ended. In the event that we have to pause a regression after releasing either an event or a perpetrator (for lack of time or an unexpected reason), the regression may be continued at that point in a subsequent session; otherwise, continue.

### Uncovering Other Events

Once the client confirms complete release of the event, we can now proceed to confirm whether any other events must be discovered and released. Ask a question such as the following:

> **Please allow your subconscious, or your inner mind, to answer the next question with the appropriate finger response: Is there any other event that must be discovered and released?**

In the event of either a "yes" or "I don't know" response to the above question, at least one more regression is required to discover and release another event. Whether the second regression occurs the same day (time permitting) or at a subsequent session, we need to be ready to change regression techniques if necessary in order to guide the client back appropriately to another event. Also, we often may not know whether the event already cleared is the ISE or the AE until after the second event is uncovered during hypnosis.

Even after confirming release of the second event at a second regression, we should still ask the question about any additional events. On occasion, the subconscious takes a client back to one or more SSEs in order to completely release a problem.

Years ago, one of Roy Hunter's hypnotherapy students had a fear of snakes. Her phobia was so intense that she was unable to even look at a picture of a snake. He employed the affect bridge in a classroom demonstration, taking her back to an incident at age three, which proved to be her ISE.

After she picked up a snake in the yard, her father panicked and told her to run for her life. She watched him use a shovel to beat the snake to a bloody pulp, resulting in her father imprinting his fear of snakes onto his daughter. Meanwhile, her older brother watched from the porch. The AE occurred only a few hours later, as her brother dropped a garden snake in her lap and said, "Snake's gonna get you! Run, run for your life!"

Her subconscious indicated more events to discover and release. The first SSE that needed to be cleared happened during grade school when her brother learned that he could terrify his sister with just a photograph of a snake. The final subsequent sensitizing event requiring release happened at a frat party in college, when her boyfriend threw a live snake around her neck as a joke. She ran out the front door screaming, running across the street and almost getting run over by a car while she threw off the snake.

After the session, she told the class that she discarded the boyfriend almost as quickly as she discarded the snake. Several weeks after the classroom session, she told the class that she was now able to look at pictures of snakes even though she retained respect for the danger of the poisonous ones.

## When All Events are Released

Whether it takes one regression or several regressions, we should be persistent until the client finally indicates that there are no further events to discover and release. When that confirmation comes from the subconscious, ask:

**Is that problem and its causes totally released now?**

Once the client answers in the affirmative, we can move into the subconscious relearning phase discussed in the next chapter. However, when the client answers the above question with either a "no" or "I don't know" response, ask what it will take to completely release the problem, and deal with what emerges. If the subconscious does not know how to obtain total release, then consider scheduling parts therapy or one of its variations (such as ego state therapy or voice dialogue) in a subsequent session.

Note that after successfully releasing all events pertaining to the cause of the problem, the third of the four primary hypnotherapy objectives is complete: *release*. We are now ready to move into Phase 4: subconscious relearning.

# CHAPTER 6

# Phase 4: Subconscious Relearning

After confirming release of the event(s) that caused the client's presenting problem, it is important to enable the subconscious to accept the desired changes. This is the fourth primary hypnotherapy objective discussed in Chapter 1.

## Why Subconscious Relearning is Important

One of the authors, Roy Hunter, learned the importance of this vital objective early in his hypnotherapy career. He used age regression to discover the cause of a smoker's inability to respond to hypnotic suggestions to stop smoking; but he forgot to complete the subconscious relearning objective after releasing the cause. We will call the client John (not his real name). During his teens, John's father caught him smoking behind the barn with a couple of friends, and humiliated him in front of those same friends.

Gestalt therapy during the regression enabled John to vicariously vent the emotions towards his father, which had remained bottled up over the years. He said, "Dad, you don't deserve the right to punish me for smoking while you stand there blowing cigarette smoke in my face. You are a hypocrite."

Responding as his father, the comment was: "Do as I say, not as I do ..." That intensified John's anger towards his father, who actually made that comment to John many times during his childhood. A rather intense dialogue continued for several minutes during the Gestalt role play, finally resulting in complete release of his father's hypocrisy. After confirming release of the event that proved to be both the ISE and AE, a happy client left Roy's office ... only to backslide within a week.

John told Roy that he was waiting at a long stoplight, watching the driver in the car next to him puffing away on a cigarette. He said, "I fantasized the taste and smell of the cigarette, and immediately wanted one out of habit. Since I always backslide whenever I quit smoking, I knew it was only a matter of time before I would fail again, so I went to the store and bought a pack."

Even though the cause of the smoking habit was discovered and released, John backslid because he still *believed* that he was a smoker. In other words, he needed to be convinced both consciously and subconsciously that he was *now a non-smoker*. After receiving post-hypnotic suggestions and imagery of his success, as well as the benefits of remaining a non-smoker, John reported lasting success a year later.

The above example demonstrates the importance of completing the fourth primary hypnotherapy objective after successful release of the cause(s) of the problem, and why we should use suggestions and imagery (and/or other techniques) to complete the relearning process.

## How to Facilitate Relearning

After confirming release of the problem and its causes, we may simply ask the following question:

> **As a result of what you have discovered and released, how will you best benefit in the here and now, and in the coming days, weeks and months?**

Most clients will answer that open-ended question with one or two empowering statements that we can use as a springboard for more suggestions and imagery. If the client uses a negative statement such as, "Well, I won't be afraid to get on an elevator anymore," we can phrase it as a positive suggestion:

> **From now on, you can easily and comfortably get on an elevator. In fact, just imagine yourself doing so right now …**

Continue with appropriate suggestions and imagery for the resolution of the client's presenting problem. Use direct and indirect suggestion, as well as imagery and Ericksonian metaphors, as appropriate for the client. If the original concern was habit control and/or motivation, we can use the client's original list of personal benefits of success (from the intake) as a guide to formulating appropriate imagery.

Years ago, one of Roy Hunter's clients was unable to make any progress during her first two sessions for weight reduction, even though she strongly desired to enjoy the benefits she listed at the first session. Age regression revealed an event during childhood when she was bullied, and her mother told her that someday she would be "big" and people would not push her around. Her subconscious interpreted big as *wide* rather than growing up; so that one event followed by her mother's authority imprint proved to be the core cause of her inability to reduce after many attempts and numerous diets. After confirming release, Roy used programmed imagery of her personal benefits that she revealed during her first session, and she was well on her way to success.

Some professionals familiar with Roy Hunter's methods employ EFT or other releasing and relearning/reframing techniques after a successful regression. For example, Katherine Zimmerman uses Emotional Freedom Techniques (see www.trancetime.com), but also recommended Roy's books when she taught professional hypnosis. While the use of EFT *alone* might not be sufficient for lasting results, several professionals have reported excellent results incorporating this technique during the relearning phase. Again, nothing speaks louder than success. Practitioners of EFT may choose to use it to enhance the subconscious relearning process if desired.

Other techniques can also be used to enhance the subconscious relearning process, including (but not limited) to NLP, whether or not they are mentioned in this book. Remember to use whatever techniques are appropriate for discovering the cause and facilitating release; because if any of the four hypnotherapy objectives are omitted, there is an increased risk of backsliding.

If a technique works, use it; but do *not* use any technique exclusively. There is no technique that is effective enough to work with all the clients all the time; so fit the technique to the client rather than vice versa.

The authors have worked with numerous clients over the years who did not enjoy lasting results when working with other hypnotists who failed to accomplish all four hypnotherapy objectives; so be sure to enable the subconscious to discover and identify the cause and release it. Then thoroughly complete the subconscious relearning process with suggestions and imagery after confirming release. Once subconscious relearning is complete, it is time to conclude the session.

# CHAPTER 7

# Phase 5: Concluding the Session

After giving suggestions and imagery for subconscious relearning, we may include some basic suggestions for general well-being (i.e., ego strengthening) as well if desired. Since a deeper trance state occurs towards the end of a long session, it is wise to use a very slow and directive re-alerting procedure (one to two minutes).

When the client first emerges from hypnosis, he/she is responsive to suggestions, so we must choose our first words carefully. This caution is rarely discussed even among experienced hypnotherapists, thus it is also rare to find it in writing. Roy Hunter mentions this caution in chapter 7 of *The Art of Hypnotherapy* (Hunter, 2010b), and Stephanie Rothman has posted an article on her website with the same warning (Rothman, 2011).

As appropriate, provide a few minutes for debriefing, and schedule the next session. Both authors normally like to see a client as least one more time after an intensive regression, and will customize that session based on the degree of progress. If the client has traveled a great distance, we advise the client to seek local follow-up as appropriate to insure continued success.

## Steps for Concluding the Session

There are three basic steps to concluding a regression session with a client:

1. Give additional ego strengthening suggestions for the client's well-being.
2. Use a slow directive re-alerting (or awakening) procedure.
3. Debrief.

It is appropriate to suggest that a client imagine feeling good and/or rested after an intensive regression session. However, it is not wise to use a rapid re-alerting technique, because some clients will have "hypnotic hangover" (such as a headache) if awakened quickly after experiencing deep trance for a length of time. The authors recommend one to two minutes of slow counting.

As previously mentioned, we must take additional care during the debriefing because most clients remain susceptible to suggestions even after the formal re-alerting. For example, one of the authors saw a smoker who said that after seeing another hypnotist to stop smoking six months earlier, the hypnotist said: "Now don't go blowing it by lighting up if you find a pack in the glovebox of your car." The client suddenly remembered that he had a pack in the glovebox, and lit up as soon as he got into his car. Needless to say, he never returned to the woman who previously tried to help him quit.

Remember that imagination is the language of the subconscious; so it is wise to reinforce the solution rather than joking about the problem. If the client had a fear of flying, we can say something like: "You will be much more comfortable next time you fly." We could also say something such as, "Isn't this amazing stuff?" After the client responds, we may simply reinforce the success mindset with additional positive suggestions for success.

Also, note that a successful regression therapy session accomplishes all four hypnotherapy objectives.

## Did You Discover and Release the Core Cause(s) and Facilitate Relearning?

A successful hypnotic regression therapy session (or series of regressions) accomplishes the four primary hypnotherapy objectives discussed in Chapter 1:

1.  Suggestion and imagery (first session without regression, then Phase 4 of regression)

2. Discover the cause (may take more than one regression)

3. Release (may take more than one regression)

4. Subconscious relearning (enhanced with suggestion and imagery and/or other techniques such as EFT or NLP)

Regression therapy is much more client centered when the hypnotherapist is competent in additional techniques beyond those covered thus far in this book. Remember that the first hypnotherapeutic step to change (post-hypnotic suggestion and imagery) becomes the final step when the others are used, whether employing regression therapy, parts therapy (or its variations) or any other technique.

If for any reason we are unable to accomplish all four hypnotherapy objectives with a series of regressions, we should consider either parts therapy (or one of its variations) or use another technique or modality such as NLP. If necessary, set your ego aside and refer the client to another professional.

## Additional Hypnotic Advice

Remember that a hypnotic regression should be the *client's* experience. In a session I (Hunter) had with a middle-aged man lacking confidence, he indicated during the intake that his problem probably started when the "inner child" was hurt as a small child. His father scolded him, breaking a glass in his face. He was familiar with John Bradshaw's work involving the importance of healing the inner child (Bradshaw, 1988).

Although I explained the importance of setting aside preconceived opinions, he still wanted to return to that specific event during HRT. Since the client writes my paycheck, I honored his request; but his subconscious resisted any abreactions and indicated that the cause was another event. That session validates the fact that often the client's preconceived opinion regarding the cause of a problem is incorrect. A second regression uncovered the correct ISE for his problem. However, the client ultimately pays your wages, whether you are self-employed or work for a clinic; so if a client insists on starting with a regression to a specific event, it is okay to honor that request. Just be aware that often there is more to discover.

Also, be conscious that regression will not work for all the people all the time, no matter which regression technique you use. More than once during Roy Hunter's initial training, he personally witnessed Charles Tebbetts changing techniques in mid-trance—switching from regression to parts, or vice versa. Tebbetts taught that the competent hypnotherapist sometimes must work by trial and error, changing techniques to adapt to the client. However, if you have not yet done a proper pre-talk on regression or parts therapy, use suggestion and imagery and schedule another session in order to be sure the client is comfortable with the technique you choose to use.

Also, do both yourself and your clients a favor by being willing to learn and use a variety of techniques, so that you may fit the technique to the client rather than the other way round. This diversified client centered approach will serve both you and your clients far better than using one primary modality.

It is also appropriate to follow up with the client after a successful hypnotic regression therapy session by either scheduling at least one additional session from one to four weeks later, or scheduling a phone consultation to find out if any more hypnotherapy is needed to help insure lasting success.

Even though this book has now covered the essential phrases and steps of HRT, no book on regression would be complete without a discussion of one of the most controversial topics in hypnosis: *past life regressions*. Regardless of your opinions, the authors hope that you will find the next chapter to be both educational and enlightening.

# CHAPTER 8

# Past Life Regressions: Fact or Fantasy?

Even as we enter the first century of the new millennium, people both inside and outside of the hypnotherapy profession still hotly debate the topic of past life regressions.

Two major religions believe in past lives (Buddhism and Hinduism). In addition, while most Christians believe that we only live once, as of 1997, Elizabeth Clare Prophet stated that there are 28 million Christians who believe in reincarnation (Prophet & Prophet, 1997). According to Rabbi Yerachmiel Tilles, Judaism also accepts reincarnation. He posted an article on the internet that states:

> Consequently, many Jews are surprised to learn, or may even wish to deny, that reincarnation —the "revolving" of souls through a succession of lives, or *"gilgulim"*—is an integral part of Jewish belief. But this teaching has always been around. And it is firmly rooted in source-verses. (Tilles, 2011)

Additionally, some Bible scholars familiar with the writings of Flavius Josephus (an ancient Jewish historian) realize that Josephus wrote about the Pharisees being believers in reincarnation, while the Sadducees rejected it. A significant number of Jewish people living during the time of Christ were Pharisees.

The reason for mentioning this is that regardless of your own views, a very significant percentage of the world's population accepts the concept of living more than once. That makes the topic very relevant to hypnotherapists around the world, even if most people in your country are skeptical of the concept of past lives.

This chapter will neither prove nor disprove the validity of past life regressions; instead, it will provide some food for thought regardless of whether the reader is a believer, a skeptic or undecided.

While it is a proven fact that clients in hypnosis may be intentionally guided into what seem to be memories of a former lifetime, stranger yet is that a past life regression (PLR) can sometimes happen spontaneously. Even clients who do not believe in former lives may, on rare occasions, trip out unexpectedly into real or imagined memories of a "past" life during what was intended to be HRT back to an event from the client's present life. Regardless of whether a hypnotherapist chooses to facilitate past life regressions, we cannot ignore the fact that a PLR can sometimes occur spontaneously. Why? This chapter will attempt to answer that question to your partial satisfaction, regardless of your personal, professional, philosophical or spiritual beliefs.

Sadly (yet true to human nature), most available information on this controversial subject either attempts to promote the theory of reincarnation or to discredit the idea altogether. Some highly educated people believe that the concept of living more than once is unscientific; yet others with medical and other advanced degrees do believe that we live more than once. For example, Brian Weiss, M.D., a psychiatrist, has written several books regarding past life regressions since facilitating a spontaneous PLR for a patient (Weiss, 1988, 1993, 1996). He also gives workshops on past life therapy (see www.brianweiss.com). Likewise, while most Christians argue vehemently against the concept on theological grounds, some ordained Christian ministers believe in reincarnation. One of them was the late Arthur Winkler, Ph.D., a former Methodist minister (and author) who was a friend of Roy Hunter. Winkler's book, *Reincarnation and the Interim between Lives* (1976), reported his findings from regressing over 8,000 individuals.

Regardless of your opinions on the PLR controversy, the authors believe that it will be worthwhile to both you and your clients for you to read this chapter. First, we will consider some possible explanations of the past life regression phenomenon.

## Possible Explanations

There are several popular theories to explain what may be taking place during a past life regression. You are free to choose the theory (or theories) which fits comfortably into the framework of your own personal and/or professional beliefs.

### Fantasy or Metaphor (False Memories)

Any competent hypnotherapist knows that hypnosis enhances one's own ability to imagine or fantasize; and this most certainly provides a logical explanation for many past life regressions: *false memory syndrome*. Such fantasies may easily spring from curiosity, fascination for a particular place or time period in history and/or identifying with a certain historical person—or they might simply be the result of a subconscious metaphor that may facilitate change in your client. There could also be other reasons for the fantasy, such as a story, movie, TV program, dream or past event that made a subconscious impact during the client's present life, even if forgotten consciously.

Additionally, any willing client (or subject) can confabulate a past life fantasy if a hypnotist uses inappropriate leading; and unfortunately, some practitioners have done this repeatedly over the years.

It is the authors' belief that numerous past life regressions facilitated by competent hypnotherapists fall into the category of fantasy or metaphor. However, it is worthwhile to consider alternative explanations, if only to be able to talk with clients who hold these beliefs.

### Soul Memories (Reincarnation)

Many believe that past life regressions prove reincarnation, as is evidenced by the many books written on the subject. Even some Christians believe that the family of Jesus was among the Essenes, who believed in reincarnation. Years ago a Jewish rabbi shared this information about the Essenes personally with Roy Hunter in order to console him on the day of his mother's funeral.

Arthur Winkler facilitated thousands of past life regressions during his life (Winkler, 1976). He studied numerous results and eventually he formed the opinion that many of them were valid. (Since there are untold millions of Christians who believe that reincarnation is in total conflict with Christianity, this is not the place to debate it.)

Brian Weiss changed his paradigm because of a spontaneous PLR that occurred during therapy with a patient. He shared this unusual journey in detail in his book, *Many Lives, Many Masters* (1988), and has written numerous books since.

Other books indicate alleged past lives as well, such as *Children who Remember Previous Lives* by Ian Stevenson (1987), and *Children's Past Lives* by Carol Bowman (1998). However, an apparent PLR or memory of the life of someone who actually lived does not necessarily prove that the individual in hypnosis was the same soul who lived those lives. There are other possible explanations.

### Soul-Tapping
The person in hypnosis may "tap into" the actual memories of another soul who lived in the past, finding those memories from the Universal Book of Life, Holy Spirit or from the Akashic records, or by telepathically reading (or channeling) actual thought patterns from the soul of another who is in spirit form.

The subconscious and/or superconscious finds something relevant for the client at the time for the person's soul growth, and we tune into and "play" the memories much like a DVD player playing a DVD, or a DVR player playing a pre-recorded cable program or movie.

Some who object to the idea of reincarnation on religious grounds may find this concept to be an acceptable explanation for past life regressions.

### Universal Consciousness
This theory is similar to the one above. The belief is that we are all interconnected through the spirit of God or Universal Consciousness,

and therefore all memories of all lives ever lived (both past and present) are instantly available through hypnosis if needed for one's own personal or spiritual growth. We can access them through Universal Consciousness, Holy Spirit, Holy Ghost, Divine Light, or Superconsciousness, Higher Self and so on; and the inner mind chooses a life to replay that relates to the client's problem. This idea is also similar to Carl Jung's archetype concept.

### Genetic Memory
Some people believe that memories may be passed on through heredity. This theory does not hold water with regressions where one remembers his/her death. Neither would it explain why memories for a particular life would continue after one's last child was conceived; nor would it explain a Japanese client regressing into an apparent Native American lifetime in the late 19th century (as happened to a client of one of the authors).

You are free to consider still other possible explanations besides these; but perhaps this gives you a starting point for opening your mind to possible explanations for those past life regressions that seem to be more than just fantasy. Even if you do not wish to choose any explanation other than fantasy, there remains the mystery of the occasional spontaneous past life regression.

## Spontaneous Past Life Regression

Whether or not you believe in past lives, on rare occasions a client might (as mentioned earlier) spontaneously "trip out" into a real or imagined past life. A spontaneous PLR can happen even when the therapist is a professional with a doctorate degree, and skeptical of past life regressions.

Using the affect bridge technique can sometimes trigger such a regression, even when that was not the intention of either the therapist or the client—and this may happen even when neither the therapist nor the client believe in past lives. This was the case with both Brian Weiss and Arthur Winkler (discussed above), whose paradigms changed because of unplanned past life regressions. Winkler also personally informed Roy Hunter that his client's spontaneous past life regression changed her life as well as his life.

If a client experiences a spontaneous PLR, stay calm. Take a deep breath and say "relax" to both your client and to yourself, in order to calm your own anxiety, since this can be picked up by the client's subconscious. If you are comfortable dealing with what emerges, guide the client through the experience. Remember to *allow* (but not force) abreactions in accordance with Phase 3 of regression therapy in order to help the client release the perceived cause of the problem, and then confirm release. Facilitate subconscious relearning as well. (Refer to Chapters 5 and 6 as necessary.) Handle it much the same as you might handle a present life regression—making sure to suggest a total return to the present day before re-alerting.

If you are not comfortable handling the spontaneous PLR, bring your client back to the present life quickly but gently; but do *not* re-alert from hypnosis just yet. Guide him/her to a safe place and ask the subconscious to disclose any possible relevancy to the present life. If you have difficulty doing this, just give some soothing post-hypnotic suggestions for peace and well-being, along with suggestions that any relevant information be dealt with at another appropriate time and place. Then, after re-alerting, ask the client to tell you how he/she feels about what happened during hypnosis.

If the client wishes to explore the real or imagined past life, you have an important decision staring you in the face. Under no circumstances should we criticize a client for regressing back too far in time. If he/she believes in former lives, then you serve him or her better with a referral to an ethical hypnotherapist who is comfortable working with past life therapy; otherwise, become more comfortable with PLR techniques yourself so that you may easily facilitate the rare spontaneous past life regression.

Years ago, a devout Lutheran who saw Roy Hunter to deal with the fear of flying experienced a spontaneous PLR, and regressed back to a real or imagined death experience. She did not believe in past lives, yet she vividly described suffocating to death. After releasing the emotions and entering the relearning phase, she said that it was not being high in the sky that she feared while flying. Rather, it was the fear of running out of oxygen in a pressurized cabin and dying again like before. Upon re-alerting, she exclaimed, "That seemed pretty real! Did I really live before this life?"

Note that this was a no-win question! To validate her experience as "real" might have caused anxiety over her religious convictions, with a possible crisis of faith and/or possible marital stress. To invalidate it as false memory could have invalidated the release from her former fear of flying. The most considerate and professional response was to give her an answer that allowed her to explore her own conclusions.

Roy's response was that it was not his place to say whether her experience was real. She could have seen a movie or heard a story as a small child, or her subconscious could simply have produced this story as a metaphor to help her. He briefly summarized the possible explanations and finished by saying, "Whether or not you really lived that life isn't nearly as important as your release from the phobia, is it?" Her release from the fear of flying was permanent. Several years later, she told Roy that she had flown over 250,000 miles since that session.

While the spontaneous PLR seems to provide an excuse for some hypnotists to offer a PLR to their clients and/or try to convince a client that the origin of a problem is past life karma, the authors judge that this is a risk to everyone concerned. At the other extreme, some clients who request a past life regression receive criticism from a therapist who is a past life skeptic. The authors believe that we should put the client ahead of our own beliefs, so please consider the ethical considerations covered below.

## Ethics (of Past Life Regressions)

We need to work within the comfort zone of the client, doing what we would want done if the roles (and beliefs) were reversed. With that in mind, we now explore the ethics of three possible basic beliefs of the hypnotherapist: past life believer, past life skeptic and undecided.

### If You Believe in Past Lives ...

It is unethical to intentionally initiate a past life regression unless your client requests it (Hunter, 2010b). Even if you believe the problem originated in a former lifetime, you risk the credibility of hypnotherapy by taking it upon yourself to force the person into a PLR unless that is what the client, of his/her own free will, chooses in advance of the trance.

Furthermore, some people may feel it is an infringement of their own beliefs if a hypnotherapist solicits their consent prior to the hypnotic session; so the client should initiate the request unless we already know for certain that the client believes in the possibility of past lives.

Each of the authors in their practices have listened to clients complain about other hypnotherapists who tried to convince them that their problems originated in past lives. Presuming that the cause of a person's problem is the result of past life karma is a grave mistake. It constitutes diagnosing with no legitimate basis. Even if both the client and the hypnotherapist believe in past lives, facilitating a PLR to look for the cause of a problem could result in false memories, which would allow the actual core cause of the client's problem to remain buried in the subconscious if the ISE occurred in the client's current life.

If a client asks your opinion on past lives, consider carefully before disclosing. In some situations, you might be taking a professional risk to tell a client that you believe in past lives—depending on the client's own beliefs. Also, remember that even a spontaneous past life regression does not prove that your client actually lived that life. Briefly summarize the possible explanations in order to help the client feel comfortable with the session. More importantly, do *not* attempt to use the spontaneous PLR experience to convert that person's belief system to match your own. Again, put yourself in your client's shoes.

Should you advertise that you practice past life therapy, you risk limiting your market of prospective clients. Should you choose to take that risk, consider the possible cost to your pocketbook as well as your credibility.

### If You Believe We Only Live Once ...
The other side of the coin is that the past life skeptic may appear as cold and insensitive if trying to convince a client that it is unscientific, un-Christian or stupid to believe in past lives. In the latter half of the 20th century, a famous trainer publicly denounced past life therapy as being unethical, prohibiting its practice for any member of the hypnosis association he founded. Roy Hunter personally heard this person *publicly* criticize past life regressions in 1990. This type of criticism hurts our profession and creates more division.

Several clients have complained to one of the authors after receiving criticism from a hypnotherapist or psychologist for believing in reincarnation. That is understandable, given that the hypnosis association referred to above banned its practice for decades.

All of us are certainly entitled to our own belief systems, and that includes our clients. However, in the opinion of the authors, we as hypnotherapists have a responsibility to do our best to work with our clients as much as possible *within the framework of their own spiritual beliefs* regardless of our own personal beliefs.

You do not have to honor a client's request for a PLR; but it is unprofessional to convince the client that past life therapy is unethical. Instead, the ethical guideline for the past life skeptic is: give the clients who request past life regressions the courtesy of tactfully referring them elsewhere *without criticizing either them or their beliefs*.

Remember that we are here to serve the client, *not* to convert clients to our own spiritual, philosophical or personal beliefs. The client's need is more important than our own personal beliefs or ego. As with the past life believer, the PLR skeptic takes a risk in sharing his/her skepticism with a client. The client who believes in past lives may take such an opinion as criticism, resulting in loss of rapport (and probable loss of a client).

We certainly do not appreciate it when prospective clients are convinced by outside prejudice to avoid hypnosis. Since we want the public to be open minded about hypnotherapy, we owe it to our clients, ourselves and our entire profession to keep an open mind about ideas we might not use in our own practice, including past life regressions. Asking others to be open minded about hypnotherapy while remaining closed minded about the potential benefits of past life therapy has a rather strange hypocritical ring in the ears of many hypnotherapists. That being said, one of the authors has met several hypnotherapists who consider themselves to be past life skeptics, but nonetheless are willing to facilitate a PLR upon request.

Even though you have no obligation to accommodate a request for a PLR, with a little experience and sensitivity you just might find yourself able to facilitate this upon request. Some of the techniques mentioned later in this chapter might also help you and your client.

### If You are Undecided ...

If you are in this group, it is easy and relatively safe to be open and honest about your undecided opinions. It is totally acceptable and professional to admit to a client that you do not know whether the experience was real or metaphoric, and the client will most likely respect your honesty.

Roy Hunter has personally told some clients, "I am not a scientist, so is it *not* my job to research the validity of past lives. Also, my opinions may or may not be correct, so it is up to you to decide for yourself. As for me, I choose to keep an open mind." Very few people can criticize this type of response as unprofessional unless they cling to very biased opinions.

Now that we have considered possible explanations and some ethical issues, it is time to look at some actual techniques that can be used to facilitate the requested past life regression.

# Techniques to Initiate a Past Life Regression

We may use the preparation phase for a PLR in much the same manner as with HRT for the present life, incorporating all the same steps, but adding the safeguard described below. However, during the pre-induction discussion, it is client centered to briefly describe the six techniques presented in this section and ask the client to choose.

The somnambulistic state provides the best probability of a successful past life regression; however, clients will often respond even in a medium depth of trance. In a light level of hypnosis there is usually too much conscious interference to allow a successful regression, although occasional exceptions occur. Thus, it is wise to endeavor to get the client deeper than 40 on the 100 to 1 scale.

As with hypnotic inductions, the ways of initiating a requested PLR are as limitless as the imagination. We will consider some of the more commonly used methods of helping a client become an explorer of real or imagined past lives. Before we begin, however, we should consider giving the client (or explorer) a safeguard.

### Building a Link to the Present (A Safeguard)

Prior to starting hypnosis, ask the client to agree to be aware of your voice at all times, and to return immediately to the present when asked to do so. Explain to them that these are the "conditions" of being a past life explorer—and that they will also be asked while hypnotized if they still agree to the "conditions." After the last step of the preparation phase, ask for an ideomotor response to indicate acceptance of the conditions. Then use one of the PLR regression techniques described below, which the client chooses before entering hypnosis.

### The Time Tunnel

The explorer enters a time tunnel of deep hypnosis, going deeper back through time. The tunnel may be lit softly with the explorer's favorite color. In addition, the client may walk or float through the tunnel, or sit on a vehicle such as a Disneyland type riverboat or similar.

Once we guide the client inside the tunnel, we may use words such as:

> As you go deeper into the tunnel, you go deeper into hypnosis—always aware of my voice. Deeper and deeper, going back ... to another time, another space ... another life, another place ... another body, another face ... the choosing of your higher mind [*inner mind, higher self, Higher Power, etc.*].
>
> *Repeat the previous paragraph if desired.*
>
> Off in the distance now is the tunnel exit, where you will come out into another time, another space ... another life, another place ... another body, another face ...
>
> You are nearing the exit now ... leaving the tunnel, and becoming more aware of where you are as I count from 1 to 3.
>
> Number 1: out of the tunnel now.
>
> Number 2: becoming more aware of anything you see, hear or feel.
>
> Number 3: BE THERE! Make a report ... What do you see, hear or feel?

At this point, we may guide the client through the regression. (See the comments on page 145 for clients who do not respond.) If the regression is purely for curiosity, there is no formal second or third phase; but be prepared for possible abreactions, dealing with what emerges.

## The Cloud Technique

The explorer can simply imagine becoming surrounded by a hypnotic mist of his/her favorite color. Then we may use words such as the following:

> As you begin drifting deeper and deeper into hypnosis, you feel lighter and lighter as though you are floating within the mist of deep hypnotic sleep ... In fact, you find it more and more enjoyable just to let yourself go, drifting into the cloud ... and you are always aware of my voice as you keep on drifting way back through time, farther and farther into hypnosis.

> Drifting way, way back ... to another time, another space ... another life, another place ... another body, another face ... the choosing of your higher mind [inner mind, higher self, Higher Power, etc.].

> *Repeat the previous paragraph if desired.*

> The cloud is slowing down, now ... slowing down and ever so gently descending down, down, down ... gently setting you down ... And as I count from 1 to 3, the cloud will vanish, allowing you to become more and more aware of where you are.

> Number 1: the cloud is beginning to disappear now.

> Number 2: becoming more aware of anything you see, hear or feel.

> Number 3: BE THERE! Make a report ... What do you see, hear or feel?

Deal with what emerges.

## The Crystal Hall Technique

Generally, the explorer must be able to visualize easily in order for this technique to be effective. The client enters a long hallway with walls and ceiling of crystals and a floor of fine marble, glass or gold. At the other end of the hall is a door with a huge, emerald doorknob. We may ask the client to enter the hall from his/her peaceful place, saying words such as:

> Now that you've agreed to the conditions, you may find the door to the crystal hall appearing. As the door opens, you may enter the hall. It may be rounded or shaped in whatever manner you wish. Its walls are covered with glittering crystals or jewels of many colors. Its floor is fine marble, glass or gold. Move your finger when you are in the hallway ...

> *Wait for response.*

> This is a hallway back through time and space ... At the end of the hall is a door opening up into another life, another place ... another body, another face ... the choosing of your higher mind [*inner mind, higher self, Higher Power, etc.*]. There is a huge emerald knob on the door, and when you are ready, you may touch the knob and the door opens ...
>
> Touch the knob now, and step through the open door ... As I count from 1 to 3, you become more and more aware of where you are.
>
> Number 1: the door closes behind you, and you become aware of where you are.
>
> Number 2: becoming aware of anything you see, hear or feel.
>
> Number 3: BE THERE! Make a report ... What do you see, hear or feel?

Note that the explorer *must* exit the hallway! If he/she fails to exit through the door on the first request, it is appropriate to make a second attempt in a more direct way. Very visual clients often want to stay in the hall after being dazzled by the beauty they create in their minds. If the client is still stuck in the hall after the second attempt to get him/her through the door, then guide him/her back to the safe place and use another regression technique.

Another variation on the above technique is to have the client enter the hallway of time, with numerous doors representing centuries; and the client selects that door which is most appropriate and beneficial to open. When the client steps through, deal with what emerges.

### The Elevator through Time
The explorer enters an elevator that descends down through the ages. Make sure the client is comfortable with elevators before using this technique.

Imagine this elevator any way you wish it to be … and as you enter, you begin to feel it moving down, taking you down deeper into hypnosis, and deeper into the past …

It's going way down now, down through the years or centuries, and you are going way down into a very deep, hypnotic sleep. The elevator is taking you way down through the ages, to another time, another space … another life, another place … another body, another face … the choosing of your higher mind *[inner mind, higher self, Higher Power, etc.]*.

*Repeat the previous paragraph if desired.*

The elevator is slowing down now, coming to a stop. As I count from 1 to 3, you become more and more aware of where you are.

Number 1: the door opens.

Number 2: step out of the elevator and be aware of anything you see, hear or feel.

Number 3: BE THERE! Make a report … What do you see, hear or feel?

If you are changing to this technique after lack of response to another, then you may ask for an ideomotor response to determine whether the client is comfortable with elevators. Once the client steps out into the past, deal with what emerges.

### The Bridge across the River of Time

The explorer crosses a meadow, noticing a river with a footbridge. It is the river of time. On the far side of the bridge is a strange mist, with a rainbow where the path enters the mist. After stepping under the rainbow into the mist, the mist clears—leaving the explorer in another time, another space and so on. Omit the mist or rainbow for the client who does not visualize well. A person who is primarily auditory or kinesthetic might prefer to hear the river or feel the handrail on the bridge, with a sense of crossing.

## Age Regression before Birth

There are those who simply take a client back by age regression (or calendar year regression) to birth and before, to the last lifetime before the current one, and then deal with what emerges. At first glance this might seem very appropriate to the novice, but there may be more than meets the eye.

It might be too limiting to the client if we use this technique unless that person asks to go back to what he/she believes to be the most recent lifetime before the present one, because there is a possibility that the information produced by the subconscious may not be where he/she needs to go. Bruce Eimer sometimes uses the following wording.

> *As I take the client back, I stop where it is clinically indicated, and ask the client to "be there" and report what is happening.*
>
> **Orient your mind back over the years, back over your lifetime to before you are born. Go way back. Imagine you are getting younger and smaller. Go back over the years. You are becoming younger and smaller. Smaller and smaller. Younger and younger. You are becoming littler. Going back over the years. Going back through the times when you are a little boy/girl. Going further back. Going back even earlier than that. You are going back to when you are a little itty bitty baby. A little itty bitty baby. And you are getting even smaller and younger. Smaller and younger. Now you are going back to before you are born, to when you are in your Mommy's stomach, in the womb. It is dark and warm and cozy and safe. And now you are going further back. Going back to when your Mommy and Daddy are together and create you, conceive you. Be there.** *[If indicated, stop and ask the client to tell you what is happening.]*
>
> **Now you are going back to before that. To before you are made. Going back to when your Mommy and Daddy decide to get together.** *[If indicated, stop and ask the client to tell you what is happening.]*

> Now go back to an earlier time. Go back to before you are conceived, before your Mommy and Daddy get together to make you, to conceive you. Going back over the years. Way, way, way back over the years. To an earlier time. To a time that has something important to do with your problem ... Be there!

## If There is No Response ...

If the explorer does not immediately answer, we may sometimes trigger responses with one or more of the following questions:

- **What do you see, hear or feel?**
- **Where are you?**
- **What's happening now?**
- **Are you inside or outside?**
- **Are you standing, seated or lying down?**
- **Is it dark or light?**
- **Is it cool, warm or comfortable?**

If there is still no response, then we may take the client back to his/her peaceful place for a moment. After additional deepening, we may then try another PLR technique.

If there is no response after two or three different techniques, there may be a reason for resistance. If this happens, we may take the client back to his/her safe place, and use open-ended questions to ask the subconscious where the client needs to go. Perhaps this person is not ready for a past life regression. Remember, we cannot force—we can only guide.

Also, note that a visual client might have an auditory past life regression, or vice versa. One of Roy's clients said, "I don't see anything ... everything's foggy." When he again asked what she could see, hear or feel, she went on to describe holding onto the rail of a ship while hearing a distant foghorn. Another client was totally blind since birth in his current life; but he had a very visual PLR, describing green hills and apple trees with bright red apples. After the session, he was amazed to remember what it was like to see in that former life.

## Guiding vs. Leading

Once the client starts responding, we must allow it to be a *client centered* experience. In other words, we allow the client to tell us what is happening rather than the other way around.

We again mention this caution because inappropriate leading seems to be far too common among practitioners who facilitate past life regressions. Metaphysical practitioners who consider themselves to be very intuitive (or psychic) are often tempted into leading rather than guiding, as hypnotherapists have observed during PLR workshops and demonstrations over the years. One well-known author (who will remain anonymous) often gives leading suggestions or asks leading questions. Doing so can result in a client fantasizing whatever he or she is asked to imagine, ending up in a therapist directed experience that is projected into the client. Such a PLR is likely to contain false memories or end up being a complete fantasy.

For example, let us say an explorer reports being on the beach. Ask, "What are you doing at the beach?" Do *not* ask if the client is swimming, as this could be perceived by the subconscious as a suggestion to do so. Asking the client if he is swimming could interfere greatly with what takes place in the mind, as there could be any number of reasons for being at the beach other than for a swim. Likewise, asking a client whether there is a boat or ship within view could also cause the subconscious to fabricate whatever is suggested.

Often the entire PLR begins as a fantasy because the facilitator says something like, "Go back to a life when you lived as a priest in ancient Egypt" and so forth. Again, do not assume. Ask the client's inner mind (God, Higher Power, Divine Wisdom, etc.) to guide the client where he/she needs to go, and you increase the likelihood of the experience being worthwhile for that client.

When one experience during a PLR is completed, we may guide the client forward or backward in time to, for example, a very important event, a happy experience or the most important day of that life. As appropriate, we may also guide the explorer all the way through the death experience to "the first moment of total peace after the transition" and ask him or her to talk about it. Throughout the entire PLR, we must make certain to avoid the temptation of projecting our own opinions into the client's experience.

A close friend of Roy Hunter saw a female "rebirthing" counselor who claimed competency with past life therapy. She told him that he was a mass murderer in another lifetime, and tried to make him abreact into feelings of guilt. When he brought himself out of trance and lectured her against leading, she tried to convince him that her intuition was very accurate because Mary, the Mother of Jesus, inspired her, and that he should continue seeing her. He refused; and after some questioning, he finally got her to admit that she had received no formal training in regression therapy. The rebirthing counselor apparently refused to believe that she was actually practicing a form of hypnotherapy. She was quite defensive, claiming that she could help him if he would invest in several more sessions.

## Past Life Abreactions

When facilitating past life regressions, we must be prepared to handle abreactions, even if the purpose was to honor a client's request simply from curiosity.

As discussed earlier, abreactions represent *emotional discharges* taking place because of subconscious perceptions of either actual remembered events or imagined events that may be based on either partial or total fantasy. Remember that even an intense abreaction could be a *distorted perception* of a real memory or a perception based on a fantasized event. In either case, the guidelines for handling abreactions are basically the same for either present life or past life regressions.

Remember to allow *but not force* the emotional discharge. It is also possible to use a variation on the informed soul/child technique as described below.

## Informed Soul Technique

This is similar to the informed child technique with a major modification. We may guide the client to his/her peaceful place, and then suggest that the client relive the situation as perceived, but with all the spiritual awareness and wisdom possible for a mature and spiritual understanding of the situation.

If he/she believes in the concept of a "higher spiritual self," then we may suggest "higher self" awareness. If the client believes in God and/or Universal Intelligence, or in the Holy Spirit, we can suggest that the Higher Power grant spiritual awareness as he/she relives the situation. We may then use Gestalt, or any other appropriate technique, to help the person get past the abreaction sufficiently to facilitate forgiveness and release.

An alternative is to guide the client to a sacred place and imagine talking to that person in spirit form. For some clients this type of Gestalt role play is faster than the traditional method. Remember to confirm release before moving on.

## Bypassing Abreactions of the Death Experience

To help a client bypass abreactions at a relived death experience, suggest:

> **Now move forward in time all the way through the transition to the first moment of total peace AFTER the transition ...**
>
> **How old was that body when it died?**
>
> **What was your life purpose?**
>
> **What was your main spiritual lesson in that lifetime?**
>
> *Wait for answers to each of the questions.*

Another way some therapists remove clients from the death experience and/or abreactions is to have them imagine observing, such as by watching it on a movie screen (as described in Chapter 5). Note that the imaginary movie screen will usually be ineffective with non-visual clients, in which case it may be necessary to have the client imagine being an invisible observer.

### Forgiveness and Release

Even in a past life regression, forgiveness and release should be included among the therapeutic objectives whenever abreactions occur. If Gestalt is not used, we may still choose other desensitizing techniques that might be appropriate for present life regression therapy. In addition, since clients who believe totally in reincarnation are often still distanced from that past life, we can sometimes facilitate a *generic release* with suggestions such as:

> **If there is any other person or situation to release from the lifetime just glimpsed, take a deep breath and think the word RELEASE as you exhale.**
>
> *Wait for response.*
>
> **Do you now forgive yourself for having carried that hurt as long as you did?**
>
> *Wait for response—verbal or ideomotor.*
>
> **Now I wish to ask your spiritual self (or that part of you most closely connected to God, Holy Spirit, or Universal Consciousness) to indicate if you are released and clear from that life ...**
>
> *Wait for response. You may now ask the client the following open-ended question:*
>
> **How can the lessons learned in that past life benefit you in your present life?**
>
> *Or:*
>
> **As a result of what you reviewed in that past life, how will you best benefit in the here and now of your current life, or the coming days, weeks and months?**

Note the wording carefully. This suggestion allows the client to derive benefit whether or not he/she perceives the regression as fantasy, reality or metaphor; because the "past life" is referred to as "that" past life while ownership is only suggested for the *present* life. This fine tuning of wording may help prevent a client from staying "stuck" for days in a perceived past life. Also, using either of the last two questions will create the opportunity for the client to verbalize whatever new insight was gained from the session, even if both you and the client believe the regression was fantasized.

In other words, we can assist *subconscious relearning* and enhance it with suggestions and imagery. What we are essentially facilitating in the final phase of PLR is a dis-identification or separation of the client's present life identity from that past life. In other words, we free the client from his/her identification with the self in the real or imagined past life, facilitating all relevant learning from that "past life memory" or "fantasy" and applying that learning to solving the client's problems in the present life.

Before re-alerting (or awakening) the client, we should ask him/her to return to the present and go to the peaceful place.

## Additional Remarks

There are numerous books written citing "case histories" as so-called proof of former lives; and conversely, there are religious writings condemning all who participate in past life regressions. (Christians should remember that Jesus was accused of doing the devil's work during his life.) There are also many scientific and secular critiques of past life regression work that dismiss as charlatan anyone who practices past life regression and frames the process as really tapping into past lives that the client/hypnotic subject has actually lived. You are free to pursue your own research if you choose and to form your own opinions. One interesting contribution from a psychiatrist who at one time was a part of the mainstream medical community is the book, *Through Time into Healing* (1993) by Brian Weiss, who also facilitates past life regression workshops. Another comprehensive book, recommended by a number of hypnotherapists as one of the best, was written by Roger Woolger, and is entitled *Other Lives, Other Selves: A Jungian Psychotherapist Discovers Past Lives* (1988).

The authors wish to conclude this chapter by stating the following: If you currently believe in past lives, please use caution in advertising past life therapy—as this invites criticism from skeptics. If you are totally against the concept, please remember to respect those who choose to maintain an open mind. If you are undecided, those who have already formed their opinions are advised to respect your open mindedness.

Regardless of our own personal beliefs, let us all remember the bottom line: If a client who believes in past lives is released from a problem after regressing into a real or imagined former lifetime, we have rendered a *valuable service*. Maybe it is time for us to change our paradigms.

# CHAPTER 9

# Unresolved Past Grief

Sometimes a client comes in with a presenting problem with a cause that is rooted in the past loss of a loved one (parent, grandparent, sibling, spouse, child, etc.). This may emerge during the trance state itself unless discussed by the client during the intake. While a more recent loss may require a referral to a grief counselor, hypnosis can be incredibly empowering when the loss was in the past.

Before discussing past grief, we will overview current grief.

## Grief, Mourning and Bereavement

Someone suffering a recent loss must actually go through the grief process; and usually some form of grief counseling is valuable to facilitate the process. The Encyclopedia of Mental Disorders (www.minddisorders.com) states:

> Grief counseling helps the individual work through the feelings associated with the loss of another, accept that loss, determine how life can go on without that person, and consolidate memories in order to be able to move forward. Grief counseling also provides information about the normal grieving process, to help individuals understand that many of the symptoms and changes they are experiencing are a normal, temporary reaction to loss.

Just these comments should be sufficient for any hypnotherapist or psychotherapist not trained in grief counseling to refer a client suffering from a recent loss. However, lest there be any doubt, consider J. William Worden's book, *Grief Counseling and Grief Therapy: A Handbook for the Mental Health Practitioner* (2009). It is a comprehensive book covering many different aspects of grief.

Worden is a fellow of the American Psychological Association and is a founding member of the Association of Death Education and Counseling and the International Work Group on Death, Dying, and Bereavement. He has also written several books on death and bereavement. As such, we should consider his opinions to be credible. Worden states that the term "grief" applies to the *experience* of one who suffers a loss, including (but not limited to) death. "Mourning" is the term applied to the *process* one goes through while adapting to the death of a loved one, while "bereavement" defines the *loss* the person is trying to accept (Worden, 2009: 17).

Anyone seriously interested in helping clients through the grief process of a recent loss should consider reading Worden's book. Nonetheless, unresolved past grief seems to be easier to work with for any hypnotherapist trained in HRT. However, while the techniques presented in this chapter have helped a number of clients over the years in resolving *past* grief, some of them would be inappropriate for anyone who has not yet grieved sufficiently for a more recent loss. Thus, it is our opinion that only a properly trained grief therapist should use any of these techniques with a client whose loss is recent. For some people that may be from one to two years; for others it might be three years or more.

Three proven techniques are presented in the next section. What to say during the Gestalt role play appears in the chapter section directly following those techniques.

## Techniques to Initiate Grief Resolution

The following techniques may not necessarily be the only ones available; but they have been sufficient over the years for Roy's clients. Make sure to have a tissue box nearby. You may either set a box of tissues next to the client before starting hypnosis, or set several tissues in the client's lap (or on the arm of the chair) before the trance. As an alternative, you may gently place tissues as needed in the client's hand during the actual session.

## Last Encounter

We may regress the client back to the last time he/she saw the departed loved one alive. After guiding the client through the encounter as it was perceived, we may then reframe it with Gestalt role play with the departed loved one. Here is a sample script:

> **Remember that in your imagination you can do anything you wish or BE anywhere you wish to be ... moving through time and space.**
>
> **As I count backwards from 5 to 1, go back to the last time you saw** *[name of departed]* **alive.**
>
> **5 ... moving back in time.**
>
> **4 ... imagine yourself being drawn back in time by your desire to see him** *[or her]* **again.**
>
> **3 ... going back to the last time you were with him** *[or her]*.
>
> **2 ... way back.**
>
> **Number 1 ... BE there! What's happening?**

From here, deal with what emerges. After the client relives the last encounter, guide him/her to the peaceful place. Then go back either to the event with present awareness and do Gestalt role play, or you may use the sacred place technique described below for the Gestalt role play. In either event, follow the guidelines discussed in the next major chapter section.

## Happy Event

We may regress the client back to a happy event with the departed loved one that took place prior to the passing of said loved one, and simply allow the client to enjoy revivifying it in their imagination. From there, we may either guide the client back to his/her peaceful place and go straight into Gestalt role play, or use the sacred place technique.

Here is a sample script:

> **Remember that in your imagination you can do anything you wish or BE anywhere you wish to be ... moving through time and space.**
>
> **As I count backwards from 5 to 1, go back in time to a VERY HAPPY EVENT with** [name of departed].
>
> **5 ... moving back in time, to a very happy time spent with him** [or her].
>
> **4 ... imagine yourself being drawn back in time by your desire to see him** [or her] **again.**
>
> **3 ... going back to a very happy time with** [name of departed].
>
> **2 ... way back.**
>
> **Number 1 ... BE there! What's happening?**

Before going into Gestalt (or using the sacred place technique), ask the client to describe the happy event. Be a good listener, as some clients will be very talkative.

## Sacred Place

We may help the client establish a sacred place if he/she believes in God or a Higher Power. Here is what you can say to start:

> **Once again, imagine you are in your peaceful place, with sights, sounds and sensations that are calm, peaceful and pleasant. Remember that you can do anything you wish in your imagination ... so from here, you can choose to EITHER allow your peaceful place to become a sacred place, OR you can go to another place anywhere in the universe that is a SACRED place. When you make your choice, move the "yes" finger.**

Once the client indicates making the choice, we may then ask the departed loved one to appear either in a healthy body or in spirit form, and continue as instructed in the next section.

While Roy Hunter gives credit to Charles Tebbetts for the first two techniques, he started using the sacred place technique purely from intuition; and he uses this more often than the first two techniques combined. Nonetheless, any of these techniques might be appropriate for most clients, except that the third one should only be used for someone who believes in God or a Higher Power (as previously mentioned). If the client is either an agnostic or an atheist, use the peaceful place instead of a sacred place.

## Facilitating Release and Resolution

When starting the Gestalt role play, it is usually wise to begin by asking the client to speak to the departed loved one. Here is a sample script to get you started:

> **Imagine that** [name of departed] **is before you now, and you may say anything you wish to say ...**

If the client fails to start speaking within 20 to 30 seconds, continue with:

> **Once again, imagine** [name of departed]**'s presence in front of you right now. Tell him** [or her]**: "What I wanted to say to you before you passed on is ..."**

When the client starts talking, allow him/her to speak as long as desired. Some clients may actually vent for several minutes, sobbing profusely. Allow the venting to continue without interfering until the client finishes saying whatever is on his/her mind that needs to be vented.

When appropriate, change roles, asking the departed loved one to respond. Here are some sample questions that you may ask during Gestalt when the departed loved one is responding to the client:

> - **What do you want** [client name] **to remember about you?**
> - **What encouragement or words of wisdom can you give to** [client name]?

- How can *[client name]* **best benefit from this inner dialogue?**
- **What else does** *[client name]* **need to do to enjoy greater happiness?**
- **What can you say to empower** *[client name]* **to release you?**
- **How can** *[client name]* **obtain release or closure?**
- **What can** *[client name]* **do to accept your departure and get on with life?**

Ask only *some* of the above questions—the ones that seem to be the most appropriate for your client. Note that the last three questions would be inappropriate for someone experiencing a recent loss; but a properly trained grief therapist might wish to consider using some of the techniques in this chapter if the client is open to hypnotherapy as a tool to heal more quickly from a family loss.

Depending on what emerges, the dialogue might go back and forth several times without the necessity of asking any of the sample questions. However, when it seems appropriate, say the following to both client and loved one:

**Is there anything else you wish to say before saying GOODBYE?**

In some instances the abreactions might be intense, especially if your client was elsewhere at the time of passing. The client might blame self and/or others for not being present to say goodbye, buying into feelings of guilt and/or anger towards someone else. This may be especially true if your client was a child who was prohibited from being with a parent (or grandparent) at the moment of death—in which case you might need to use Gestalt therapy with the person(s) who prevented your client from seeing the loved one at the time of passing.

One of Roy's former students had carried both anger and grief since childhood because of the passing of her grandfather. She wanted to see him one last time, but a nurse stopped her from entering the hospital room. After waiting outside the room for several minutes, she got the bad news, and was never able to overcome her bitterness towards the nurse until that session. First, Roy took her back to her last encounter with her grandfather to relive it in her imagination. Next, he regressed her to when the nurse kept her outside the room; and then he had her do Gestalt role play with the nurse. The abreactions were quite intense; but after she finally released the negative emotions, she was finally able to let go of the former grudge towards the nurse that she had carried for decades. Roy then took her to the peaceful place for Gestalt role play with her grandfather. The result was a personal breakthrough.

In some instances, the client might carry anger towards the person who passed on simply because he/she is no longer in the client's life. One of Roy Hunter's clients had to forgive a parent for passing away during her childhood and leaving her with an abusive mother. Without a husband to abuse, the mother used her daughter as a target for much of the abuse previously directed towards the client's late father. During the Gestalt, while playing the role of her father, she said: "I know your mother was abusive, and that was the hardest part of leaving you because I wanted to continue protecting you. But it was my time, so you must forgive me and release me." Although there was more dialogue than disclosed above, the client was much more empowered after the session.

## Other Comments

If you google "grief and hypnotherapy" over two million results appear. The listings on the first few pages show hypnotherapists advertising that they help with grief, and some websites simply offered MP3 downloads and CDs. Entering "grief and therapy" on Google pulled up almost 20 million results. The first few pages of the second search promote books as well as websites of grief counselors.

The person experiencing grief for a recent loss that he or she cannot process on his or her own should consider seeking competent grief counseling. Caution should be exercised in purchasing and using a generic CD or mp3 as advertised on the internet. Individualized help is usually more effective than utilizing a one size fits all tape or CD. Many CDs for processing and overcoming grief are adaptations of Elizabeth Kubler Ross's 5 stages of loss model (Kubler-Ross and Kessler, 2007).

However, in our clinical experience, this model does not apply for everyone all of the time. In our opinion, J. William Worden's (2009) book is a worthwhile read for clinicians.

With unresolved past grief, we believe that you will find the techniques mentioned in this chapter to be far more helpful than the exclusive use of hypnosis scripts. However, some unresolved grief clients might benefit from additional help and creative interventions. For example, one of Roy's clients wrote a letter to the soul of a late parent. He then signed it, prayed over it and burned it as a metaphor of release. According to the client, it worked.

In rare instances, parts therapy might be employed if the client feels an inner conflict about letting go. In addition, be aware that parts therapy itself sometimes brings up unresolved past grief. In 1999, Roy facilitated a session that was recorded in front of a live audience. The cause of the volunteer's problem related to guilt originating from a fatal auto accident some years earlier that resulted in her mother's death. The Gestalt role play was life changing for the hypnotherapist who volunteered. This case history is summarized in *Hypnosis for Inner Conflict Resolution* (Hunter, 2005).

Roy also worked with a woman for confidence and self-esteem, only to discover that the ISE of her confidence problem was her daughter's suicide four years previously. While the techniques in this chapter could have helped her release that event, the problem was compounded by the woman's loss of her son just months before the session. She was referred for grief therapy.

Conversely, another one of Roy's clients with a self-esteem problem had carried guilt since childhood when his brother was killed in an auto accident. He felt that he should have been the one to pass on instead of his brother, whom he admired. Two of the techniques presented in this chapter enabled the man to finally release his guilt and come to peace with his brother's passing.

An unusual case happened during one of Roy's classes when a hypnotherapy student asked if unresolved past grief therapy could help get over the loss of a beloved pet. Even though it seemed awkward to have the student do Gestalt role play with an imaginary animal, the result of that experimental session was successful.

In addition to the use of hypnotic techniques to help clients resolve past grief, the authors believe that much research can be done utilizing hypnotherapy as an adjunct for grief counselors to help people who are still grieving for a recent loss.

# CHAPTER 10

# Post Traumatic Stress Disorder

Every professional hypnotherapist, counselor, psychologist and physician knows about post traumatic stress disorder (PTSD), although not everyone knows how to treat it safely and effectively. The Mayo Clinic defines PTSD as follows:

> Post-traumatic stress disorder (PTSD) is a mental health condition that's triggered by a terrifying event. Symptoms may include flashbacks, nightmares and severe anxiety, as well as uncontrollable thoughts about the event. (www.mayoclinic.com/health/post-traumatic-stress-disorder/DS00246)

By clicking on "Symptoms" one reads that symptoms of PTSD include: flashbacks (for minutes or even days at a time), upsetting dreams, emotional numbness, avoiding activities previously enjoyed, hopelessness, problems with memory and concentration, and difficulty maintaining close relationships. Additional symptoms may include irritability or anger, overwhelming guilt or shame, self-destructive habits (drinking, etc.), insomnia, being startled or frightened easily, and/or hearing or seeing things that are not there.

Unfortunately, given all of the terror in the world, PTSD is a common disorder. While only about 1% of the general population suffers from PTSD (Kinchin, 2011), about 20% of veterans are impacted by the condition (Schimelpfening, 2008). The Pentagon reports that in 2007, the number of troops suffering from post traumatic stress disorder was up 50% (Jelenik, 2008). The article by Pauline Jelenik also states that many more veterans might be keeping their illness a secret. In light of this, perhaps the true percentage of the total population suffering from this condition might be higher than 1%; but even if the original estimate is correct, including veterans there would still be over three million people in the United States alone who need help overcoming the emotional devastation of PTSD.

You may wonder what the difference is between PTSD and a "normal response" to trauma (which competent hypnotherapists can clear with HRT). The Harvard Medical School help guide (www.helpguide.org) contains an article by Melinda Smith and Jeanne Segal that describes the difference:

> After a traumatic experience, the mind and the body are in shock. But as you make sense of what happened and process your emotions, you come out of it. With post-traumatic stress disorder (PTSD), however, you remain in psychological shock. Your memory of what happened and your feelings about it are disconnected. In order to move on, it's important to face and feel your memories and emotions. (Smith & Segal, 2011)

They also state that the traumatic events that lead to PTSD are usually so overwhelming and frightening that they would upset anyone.

As a clinical psychologist, I (Eimer) have treated many people over the years who suffered with PTSD. It has been my experience that if people suffering an acute reaction to stress (i.e., soon after an extraordinary life threatening event that has been experienced either first hand or vicariously) receive early and appropriate intervention (e.g., critical incident stress counseling), they can often be saved years of severe distress and dysfunction. Unfortunately, in most cases, people who have experienced critical incidents do not received appropriate early interventions and their acute post traumatic stress is often compounded by stressors emanating from supervisors, administrators, company policies, community and societal responses, the news media, relatives, neighbors, friends and so on (condemnation, negative publicity and judgments, shaming, shunning, gossip, rejection, unreasonable administrative demands from superiors at work that either prescribe unhealthy changes or prohibit healthy changes, etc.). These stressors raise the PTSD survivor's anxiety levels and anxiety related symptoms such as hyper-vigilance, guilt, intrusive thoughts and images including flashbacks, nightmares, affective blunting, social withdrawal, activity avoidance and dissociation. These clusters of symptoms unabated can eventually lead to severe depression.

Over time (typically months), a normal acute stress reaction evolves into an acute case of PTSD. At this point, it is still amenable to efficacious treatment. However, if not treated within this window, the PTSD reaction symptoms begin to spread and generalize to greater and greater aspects of the survivor's life, and a full blown chronic PTSD syndrome develops.

Although technically classified as an anxiety disorder by the American Psychiatric Association's DSM-IV (APA, 1994) (anxiety is a prime component of the disorder), PTSD is essentially a dissociative condition. As Smith and Segal (2011) observe, the mind, in response to the enduring shock of a terrifying event, disconnects the survivor's memory of what happened from his/her feelings about it. In order to heal psychologically and emotionally, the survivor must face and feel his/her memories and emotions, and in the process integrate them. Thus, effective psychotherapy for PTSD entails confronting, reviewing and reliving—mentally and emotionally—the traumatic memories, and then reframing them.

As discussed in detail by Spiegel and Spiegel (2004), people who are highly hypnotizable also score high on measures of dissociation; and people with PTSD score high on measures of hypnotizability and dissociation. Hypnosis is essentially a controlled state of dissociation and, as such, it is especially effective as a treatment tool in doing psychotherapy with people suffering from PTSD.

The hypnosis tool is invaluable in helping the client lift *repression* and *denial* through the following processes: *condensing* the essence of the traumatic experience; *uncovering* and *confessing* one's feelings about the experience and one's role in it (these feelings often include shame, guilt and anger); *normalizing* those feelings; and putting the memories and feelings into a new more adaptive and functional perspective (i.e., *reframing*) (Spiegel & Spiegel, 2004).

The essence of a generic treatment plan that incorporates hypnosis in the treatment of PTSD is to use HRT to regress the client back to the traumatic incident (TI) which is identified as the ISE. Then, following the principles of HRT delineated above, the TI is relived, the emotions are released and the client's interpretation of the significance of the TI in terms of what it says about the client's self is reframed. Then, appropriate suggestions and imagery are delivered to seal, or fix in place, the client's new learning in his/her subconscious and conscious mind.

## Causes of Post Traumatic Stress Disorder

The Mayo Clinic website (cited above) states that anyone can develop PTSD after going through (or vicariously learning about) an event that causes intense fear, helplessness or horror. Not everyone responds to an event in the same way, so doctors are not sure why some people get it while others do not. By clicking on "Causes" in the Mayo definition, it states that a complex mix of the following factors can make a person more vulnerable to developing PTSD:

- Your inherited mental health risks, such as an increased risk of anxiety and depression.

- Your life experiences, including the amount and severity of trauma you've gone through since early childhood.

- The inherited aspects of your personality—often called your temperament.

- The way your brain regulates the chemicals and hormones your body releases in response to stress.

Typical treatments recommended by numerous sources include medication, psychotherapy, hypnosis and EMDR. The U.S. Department of Veterans Affairs states that, at the current time, cognitive-behavioral therapy appears to be the most effective type of counseling for PTSD (United States, Department of Veterans Affairs, 2007). Hypnosis is a tool that makes CBT more powerful by harnessing the power of the subconscious and integrating the client's emotions and imagination.

As such, hypnosis reduces the time it takes to do CBT with clients suffering from PTSD (Zarren & Eimer, 2002).

Additionally, because a client cannot be in a truly relaxed state at the same time that he/she is in an uncomfortable emotional state, the hypnosis tool is invaluable for its power to induce relaxation states (Zarren & Eimer, 2002). Pairing relaxation with the anxiety triggered by traumatic memories is the essence of pioneering psychiatrist Joseph Wolpe's technique of systematic desensitization (Wolpe, 1973).

Hypnosis is also a focusing technique and excels in helping PTSD clients focus and concentrate on memories, thoughts and images they have been avoiding, so that this material can be reprocessed.

In the first half of the 20th century, PTSD was common among veterans of war, and was called *battle fatigue, combat stress reaction* or *shell shock*. After both the First and Second World Wars, hypnosis was often used to help combat veterans because of its more rapid results. We may verify this fact through a number of sources. An excellent manual and casebook on the use of hypnosis to treat Second World War soldiers suffering from "war neurosis", "combat stress reaction" or combat PTSD is *Hypnotherapy of War Neuroses* (1949) by the late John Watkins, who was also the co-author of *Ego States: Theory and Therapy* (Watkins & Watkins, 1997).

## Post Traumatic Stress Disorder and Hypnotherapy

Hypnotic techniques for the treatment of post traumatic conditions were frequently employed by the clinical pioneers of the end of the 19th century and by military therapists treating soldiers during the wars of the 20th century (Spiegel & Spiegel, 2004). In the past 30 years, hypnosis has been effectively employed with survivors of sexual assault, accidents and other traumas. Hypnosis as a treatment tool can be effectively integrated into psychotherapy with traumatized clients. The work of Spiegel and Spiegel (2004) indicates that individuals with PTSD frequently demonstrate high hypnotizability, which is not surprising since PTSD is essentially a dissociative condition, even though it is classified as an anxiety disorder by the American Psychiatric Association's diagnostic bible, the DSM-IV.

Hypnosis has proven to be an effective treatment tool for both authors in addressing and ameliorating the symptoms associated with PTSD. Eimer has found that hypnosis and HRT have been effective for helping clients with PTSD modulate and integrate their memories and other intrusive symptoms of trauma (e.g., flashbacks, intrusive thoughts and images, nightmares), for reducing anxiety and hyper-vigilance, and helping clients gain control over their dissociative symptoms.

Eimer has been using hypnosis and HRT for helping people recover from PTSD for over 20 years. HRT provides a vehicle for accomplishing safe reliving, abreaction, emotional reframing and ultimately desensitization. HRT does not require full exposure if the client cannot tolerate a full abreaction or an implosive experience—we can titrate the intensity of the client's exposure to the material. In any case, we can safely take the willing and collaborative client forward onto the pathway to health by helping the client reframe his/her experiences so that he/she can feel safe in the present and become more functional again.

On one level the symptoms of PTSD are caused by an associational learning of emotions which is a classical or respondent conditioning paradigm (Hall, 1976) . Essentially, the initial and subsequent sensitizing events cause "one-trial learning," and stimulus cues associated with these sensitizing events, over time, generalize to more and more aspects of the PTSD survivor's life (Zarren and Eimer, 2002). This is similar to the concept of "state dependent learning" discussed by Rossi (1993) and Rossi and Cheek (1994).

While HRT can certainly help a motivated client suffering from post traumatic stress disorder, the authors recommend that any therapist who is not trained in the specifics of PTSD either refer the client to a therapist who is, or get additional training and education in the unique aspects of PTSD and its treatment. That being said, the authors also believe that anyone already trained in treating people who suffer from PTSD would be doing both themselves and their clients a favor by becoming trained in hypnotherapy and hypnotic regression therapy.

# CHAPTER 11

# Hypnotic Regression Therapy Applications and Case Summaries

Most professionals who read hypnotherapy books find it helpful to read both applications and case histories, so we have decided to devote one chapter discussing HRT applications and summarizing interesting regression sessions. The two sections are written by each of the authors.

## Some of Bruce Eimer's Applications in Working with Chronic Pain and Post Traumatic Stress Disorder

Here is a sampling of specialized applications that have passed the test of time.

### Self-Efficacy Technique

This technique can experientially help a client with chronic pain realize that he/she can develop control over the pain. Because the client has the power to make it go up, he/she also has the power to make it go down. In other words, the cause of the problem can also become the cure. It uses the first step in the affect bridge, which in this instance is actually a *somatic bridge*. Say to the client:

> You have had this physical pain that has held you back and stopped you from feeling comfortable and enjoying your life. Today we are going to work on diminishing and neutralizing every aspect of this pain that you no longer need. That's right. In a moment I am going to count from 1 to 5 and those painful physical sensations that you don't like, that make you *[insert symptoms]*, that make you feel bad, that have everything to do with why you are here today, come up strong and powerful.

1. And now your attention goes to the physical pain in your body that you want to get rid of, that makes you [insert symptoms].

2. Coming up more and more, these physical sensations that have everything to do with why you are here today.

3. Coming up stronger and stronger, more and more powerful. I can tell that you've connected to it either consciously or subconsciously because [insert reasons].

4. Coming up stronger and stronger.

5. There it is coming up stronger and stronger ...

6. There it is. Now let yourself stay focused on the sensations. Because you made them stronger through the power of your mind, you can also make them weaker, and make them diminish through the power of your mind.

7. And now your attention goes to that physical pain in your body that you want to get rid of, that makes you [insert symptoms].

8. Coming up more and more, these physical sensations that have everything to do with why you are here today.

9. And now these pain sensations are going down and becoming weaker and weaker, softer and softer, becoming less and less. I can tell that you've connected to it either consciously or subconsciously because [insert reasons].

10. The pain sensations are getting weaker and weaker.

11. There, they are coming up softer and softer. And you are feeling more and more comfortable.

## Somatic Bridge

We now move on to doing regression using the somatic bridge. I say to the client:

> Now recognize that these pain sensations are connected to the first time in your life that you felt this way. These pain sensations are actually a bridge to the past. So, now, as I count from 5 down to 1 let yourself go back to the first time in your life when you felt that these pain sensations had become a big problem. And at the count of 1, you will step into the picture as if it is happening all over again. Touching your forehead as I count ... 5 ... and now going back to the first time when you felt that the pain was too important, a really big problem. 4 ... drifting back, floating back in the magic of the mind ... 3, 2, 1 ... BE THERE!

We then continue with Phases 3 through 5 of HRT.

## Doing Ideomotor Analysis

The following protocol is adapted from the work of David Cheek (Cheek, 1993; Cheek & LeCron, 1968; Rossi & Cheek, 1994) and Ewin and Eimer (2006). It is based on the following assumptions which are explained to the client:

> At one time in the past, your now chronic pain was acute and functional. It helped you to survive a physical insult or threat to your body. Some time after the original insult occurred, that pain began to feel just too important. It persisted beyond the point where you would have expected it to go away. It didn't go away, and you worried if it would ever go away. Your anxiety and worry became associated with the pain. When the pain didn't go away, it created more anxiety and stress. You are now tired of being in pain. You want to feel better. You want to get well.

> In order for you to feel better, these old thoughts, feelings and experiences need to be uncovered and reviewed. The subconscious negative ideas that have outlived their usefulness have to be changed, so that you can start to think and feel differently about what happened then and what is happening now. Once you do this, you will accept the idea that you no longer need all of that pain. The pain at one time served an important signaling function that assured your survival. At that time in the past,

you needed the pain to survive, AND you did survive. The pain served its purpose. Now, you are alive, and you no longer need all of that pain.

I'm going to guide you in searching your inner mind, your feeling mind, for answers to certain questions about the psychological factors that could be maintaining your pain. Concentrate on the fingers on your non-dominant hand and let them do the talking. After I ask your inner mind each feeling question, let your fingers answer what your feelings are, "Yes," "No" or "I'm not ready to answer." Each time you answer a question with your feelings, you will go deeper and deeper into self-hypnosis.

The very first thing we need to do is to ask your inner mind, your unconscious, if it feels okay to do this. So please answer with your fingers: Is it all right for me to help you with this pain problem?

*If "yes":*

Okay, your unconscious has given you the go-ahead. So, let us proceed to explore the keys to your persistent pain so that we can address and change them, and unlock the door to pain relief and comfort ...

The therapist then goes through an ideomotor exploration and analysis with the patient of each of the seven psychodynamic causes or "keys" to psychosomatic symptoms as described earlier.

### Body Lights Imagery

Ernest Rossi and David Cheek (Rossi & Cheek, 1994) developed a hypnotic imagery technique for relieving painful symptoms. The following is a step-by-step adaptation of their approach to HRT. After hypnosis is induced, say to the patient or client:

Imagine standing in front of a full-length mirror and seeing tiny colored lights in different parts of your body. These colors represent physical sensations, including comfort and pain. Your index finger on your non-dominant hand will lift up when you can see the total picture and then your finger will relax. *[Wait for finger signal.]*

Now, scan your entire body and note what each colored light that captures your attention stands for. Select the least painful body part to begin doing some therapeutic work. Let your inner mind go back to a time when that body light stood for something other than pain. When you are there, back at a time when that body part stood for something other than pain, your index finger will lift up and then relax. *[Wait for signal.]*

Okay. Be there. How old are you? Are you inside or outside? Alone or with other people? What's happening? What are you doing? What are you feeling? What are you thinking? *[Continue with the inquiry as appropriate.]*

Now move forward in time to the first moment when that light first began to stand for pain. Your index finger will lift when you arrive at that moment and then that finger will relax. *[Wait for signal.]*

Okay. Be there. How old are you? Are you inside or outside? Alone or with other people? What's happening? What are you doing? What are you feeling? What are you thinking?

*Continue with the inquiry as appropriate and then ask:*

Now please answer with your fingers. Is there any good reason now why you have to continue having pain in that body part?

*If the answer is "yes," it is important to explore the reasons. If the answer is "no," then ask:*

Now that you are aware of what is happening, is your inner mind willing to let you turn off or turn down that light, and with it that pain, and continue the healing process?

*If the answer is "no," ask:*

What stands in the way?

*If the client's inner mind is not willing to allow the pain to be turned off or down, you will need to explore with the client the factors that stand in the way of pain relief. You will most likely need to regress the client to the time when that decision was made.*

*If the client's inner mind is willing to allow the pain to be turned off or down, do a future progression by saying:*

**Go ahead now and imagine a future time when you are no longer suffering from pain in that body part. When you are there, your index finger will lift and then relax, and you will see the month, day and year as though written on a chalkboard right in front of you. Now be there. Tell me how old you are. Tell me what's happening.**

*Review with the client what transpired that helped him/her to get well. Use this report from the client to construct suggestions and images to deliver to imprint new learning and positive expectations for pain relief in the future.*

Repeat the above steps for other more painful body parts so that you gradually work your client up a sort of hierarchy of increasingly painful body parts so that he/she can get to feel more comfortable in more body locations.

### LeCron's "Control Panel of Light Switches"

Another great technique that I have used often is described by Leslie LeCron (1964) and involves asking the client to visualize a control panel of light switches with a different colored light bulb above each switch. Each switch goes to a different part of the body. The therapist asks the client:

**Visualize the area of your body that you want to work with. Now imagine a control panel of light switches with a different colored light bulb above each switch. The index finger on your non-dominant hand will lift up when you get this image and then the finger will relax.** *[Wait for finger signal.]*

Good. Now locate the switch that is connected to the area of your body that you have chosen to work with now. This switch controls the sensations in that body part. That switch sends nerve impulses from your brain down to that part of you and from that part back up to your brain. When you lock in this image, your non-dominant index finger will lift up and then relax.

*Wait for finger signal. Then ask:*

**What color is the light above that switch?**

*Then say:*

Now, turn this one switch off, and see the colored light above the switch go out. It may go out right away, or it may get dimmer and dimmer before it goes out completely. You may also hear the click of the switch as you turn the switch off. You may see the light go out, hear the switch go off or both. You may or may not immediately have a sensation of numbness or diminished sensation in the area you are working with. What is most important is to experience the diminished discomfort AND increased comfort first at an unconscious or inner level. You will know that this is happening because the index finger of your non-dominant hand will lift up and then relax as a signal.

By repeating this exercise on your own, you will experience greater comfort on a conscious level. It is important that you take the time to practice this exercise because, by doing so, you are conditioning your inner mind to be less sensitive to pain. The more you practice this exercise, the better you become at using this method to diminish your discomfort. Your success in using this exercise will also depend on your mental attitude. Doubts on your part will only impede your ability to get it to work and to get relief. Skepticism prevents self-suggestion from taking root, while positive belief promotes your ability to accomplish something worthwhile.

## Age Regression to Safe and Comfortable Times

I often age regress my pain management clients to times when they felt safe and comfortable and strong. I then have them "imprint on" (i.e., fix in place in their unconscious mind) the good feelings and body sensations they are experiencing, as well as any specific physical movements and activities associated with these good feelings and sensations. When I then age progress the client forward in time (i.e., back into the present), I suggest that the client will bring with him/her "these feelings and body sensations" and I say:

> You will find yourself unconsciously feeling this way now and even moving your body in ways that are safe and comfortable like you did back then, but your unconscious mind will only let you move in ways that are appropriate for you now. You will find it impossible to move in ways that are not safe or that could cause any re-injury.

## Split Screen Technique

This technique facilitates isolation of the components of specific traumatic memories and titrated exposure to their contents. In working with a female client who had been raped after she had agreed to go with a man she had met in a bar to another bar, I was able to help her reprocess each memory in the sequence of events leading up to the rape before she reprocessed the rape itself and its aftermath. Following the procedure described by Spiegel and Spiegel (2004), after the client attained an adequately deep level of hypnosis, I said the following:

> You are safe here in my office. Using the power of your mind and the tool of hypnosis to control what you focus your attention on, I'd like you to imagine a giant flat screen TV in front of you. Now project the first thing that happened on that screen— meeting X at the bar. Recognize that you are in control now. You can adjust the size of the image, the color, the clarity and contrast, the brightness and the audio or sound volume. You can even turn the TV off if you wish to. You can also play, fast forward, pause, stop and rewind the movie. So, go ahead and

> **run the first thing that happened on that screen and signal with your "yes" finger once you have started playing the scene.**
>
> *I waited for the finger signal and then said:*
>
> **Good, now tell me what you are watching ...**

This procedure was followed in turn for each memory in the sequence leading up to the actual rape. When indicated, the client was then told to divide the viewing screen in half. On the left half of the screen, the client first projected the man's face as he initially "worked her up" as a victim at the bar. On the right half, she projected an image of herself ignoring him and communicating her disinterest. Continued processing revealed that the man was very convincing and seductive and that he appeared to the client to be a safe and sympathetic person who was genuinely interested in her. Each piece in the sequence of events leading up to the rape was processed in this manner. Sinister parts were projected onto the left half of the screen and efficacious and responsible aspects of what the client did, knowing what she knew at the time, were projected onto the right half. This reprocessing enabled the client to realize that she had not acted as stupidly and as recklessly as she had blamed herself for acting, and that in fact, she had been taken in by an expertly smooth con man. Once the client was helped to reframe her self-perception from *stupid victim* to *unfortunately duped*, she was more amenable to forgiving herself and also emotionally releasing the perpetrator so that she could finally "file the memory away" and move on with her life.

## Some of Roy Hunter's Sessions

The sessions in this section span a period of time from late 1983 through 2011. In order to help protect client confidentiality, all names are changed as well as personal details as appropriate.

### Getting In Over Her Head

Anne was a professional woman who saw me for fear of deep water. While she was easily able to float or swim in water up to four feet deep (shoulder deep), she was unable to even walk near the edge of water that was five feet or deeper.

To make matters even more illogical, she could easily swim across the width of the swimming pool several times without touching the bottom, simply because her mind accepted the fact that she could stop swimming at any time and touch bottom with her feet. However, even though she consciously knew of her ability to swim across the width without touching bottom, the mere thought of "getting in over her head" created a state of panic.

The affect bridge technique took her back to age ten, when she and her older sister were swimming in a lake. Her sister wanted to race her to a platform about 50 yards from shore.

After her sister gained a good lead, a bully dunked Anne. The water was too deep for her to find bottom and jump back up, and she thought she would drown while fighting with the bully for dear life during precious seconds that seemed like an eternity. She finally reached the surface just in time to avoid inhaling water. While the bully laughed, she cried in anger and terror before the bully pushed her under a second time, compounding her fear. This one event at the lake turned out to be a combination of both the ISE and the AE.

I took her to her peaceful place and used the informed child technique. During the Gestalt role play, she vented considerably towards the bully before releasing him. Her subconscious indicated that no release was necessary towards her sister, who was simply too far away to help during the incident. During the relearning process, I asked her to imagine swimming across the pool at the depth level of four feet, then five feet and then nine feet.

Anne told me during the debriefing that it was amazing to realize than one childhood trauma could become the cause of a problem that lasted for many years. She let me know a month later that she did exactly as I suggested: she swam across the pool at a depth of nine feet.

## Claustrophobic Regresses to a Box

Bill had an intense fear of closed spaces. He was awaiting an MRI scan later that month, and experienced considerable stress and fear regarding the procedure. Before facilitating the regression session, I taught him the peaceful place meditation and helped him install a trigger for inner peace.

When it was time for the regression therapy, the strong emotion he felt resulted in a very quick response to the affect bridge technique. I asked, "Where are you?" He said he was in the living room, looking at a big empty TV box next to the couch. While his father was installing the new television, his older brother, Roger, tricked him into getting inside the box.

As soon as little Billy got inside the box, Roger closed the lid and sat on top, trapping Billy inside. He pleaded with Roger for over ten minutes to let him out. That seemed like an eternity to the six-year-old, who sat in darkness while hearing both his brother and father laughing at the incident.

The Gestalt was quite intense, as Bill verbalized the years of hurt resulting from his older brother's prank. After forgiving Roger, he also needed to vent anger towards his father for laughing rather than stopping the incident. Release was confirmed, followed by subconscious relearning. Nothing else needed to be discovered and released, so this one event proved to be the ISE and AE combined.

Two weeks later, Bill told me that he used his peaceful place meditation during the MRI, maintaining comfort; and he was surprised when the procedure seemed to end quickly because of the time distortion experienced during his self-hypnosis.

## Self-Esteem

Carol felt unworthy of success and seemed to sabotage herself whenever she started to succeed in her career after leaving a bad marriage. Two other therapists tried to help her, but both were into "inner child" work with the assumption that all problems originate in childhood.

The first, a hypnotherapist, tried traditional age regression, which failed. The second, a counselor, asked her to describe one of her most painful childhood events during the intake. He then used regression to a specific event that he believed was the cause, which proved to be irrelevant to the problem. Carol felt like the second therapist emotionally violated her by forcing her to vividly remember an event she had long ago forgiven and wanted to keep forgotten.

After devoting a session to learning self-hypnosis to manage stress, the affect bridge technique resulted in her going to an event during her thirties when she was fighting with her former spouse. She exclaimed during the heated argument, "I'm going to be successful whether you stay with me or not." His response was, "You'll never succeed, because you don't deserve success!"

After clearing this event with Gestalt role play, which proved to be the ISE, the subconscious revealed that another event had to be cleared. The AE happened many months later when her husband physically attacked her, and she chose to separate rather than remain married.

Within five years of her HRT sessions, she received national recognition in her profession for her success.

## A Smoking Cessation Success Story

Jim wanted to stop smoking; but self-doubts about his ability to stop the habit became magnified after several serious attempts that failed, including hypnosis. Worse, a hypnotist he saw told him that his failure was because he did not really want to quit, otherwise he would have responded to the "proven" technique and suggestions given during hypnosis.

So now my new client not only kept the smoking habit, but another so-called professional had added guilt to Jim's inability to stop smoking by planting an unconscious iatrogenic suggestion that he could not stop smoking!

As I suspected, my client failed to respond to the benefits approach of imagining his benefits from stopping; but that first session successfully increased his motivating desire to successfully become a non-smoker. Also, I let him know that it might take three or four sessions to help him reprogram his subconscious into a non-smoking mindset; so he was ready when it was time to discover the cause of his problem.

There was insufficient emotion involved to use the affect bridge technique, so instead I employed age regression. He stopped me in his early teens, when a friend convinced him to smoke because it would make him "more mature." His father caught him smoking, and harshly reprimanded him for doing so. The Gestalt was colorful because his father also smoked; but release of the event was confirmed after Gestalt both with his friend and with his father.

This proved to be the ISE; but his subconscious indicated that more had to be discovered and released. The second regression resulted in his going to his 18th birthday, when his father said, "You are now a legal adult; and if you wish to smoke, you have my permission." The approval of his father (who smoked) was an authority imprint that proved to be Jim's AE. His subconscious perceived it as his father's endorsement that smoking and adulthood go together, just as his friend had told him two years earlier.

Although Jim's success lasted at least 18 months, I lost contact with him after that. It is my opinion that if he ever backslid after my last contact with him, it was through his own volition.

### A Flying Mistake
Mike had a fear of flying that caused him to either drive or take the train whenever traveling. His wife dreamed of a vacation in Hawaii, and insisted on flying because she did not have sufficient vacation leave to go by boat.

Because he was an "analytical resister," he failed to get past a light level of trance at the first session. I taught him the peaceful place meditation and gave him a CD with instructions to listen to it at least every other day until the second session.

The second session preceded his trip by only three days, so Mike wanted it to be his last session with me because of a tight schedule. I used almost every deepening technique that I teach in order to help him get deep enough for a successful regression; but over half of his session time had evaporated by the time his "yes" finger signaled that he was deeper than 50 on the 100 to 1 scale described in Chapter 3. However, even after responding to three hypnotic convincers with additional deepening, he resisted going deeper than 40. I used the affect bridge (which often works above 40 because emotions access the right brain), but he failed to respond to the affect bridge.

Since I was running out of time, I switched to age regression even though he failed to go deeper than 40. That proved to be a mistake, because when he stopped me at age six, he spoke in the past tense rather than the present tense. Two attempts to get him to revivify (re-experience the event in his imagination) failed, because he brought himself up out of hypnosis by saying, "This isn't working ..."

I tell my students that I am willing to share my learning experiences as well as my successes so that they do not have to reinvent the wheel. The better part of wisdom would have been to devote the rest of the session to deepening him as much as possible, with post-hypnotic suggestions to attain the same depth easily at the next session, and then insist that he return one more time before his flight to Hawaii.

A month later, Mike called to tell me that his flight was not as upsetting as the last one because he had used his peaceful place meditation. However, I believe his flight could have been much more comfortable if he had allowed himself to go deep enough for me to help him release the cause of the problem.

This flying mistake occurred within three years of writing this book, making it fresh in my mind. Also, this is another example of why I emphasize the importance of getting a client deep enough before initiating a hypnotic regression.

### Dealing with What Emerges

Ken required an imagery technique for his regression; but something surprising happened during the imagery of the hallway of time. A woman stopped him in the hallway, preventing him from entering a door.

Instead of asking him how he could get past the woman, I asked, "Who is she?" My client started sobbing immediately, telling me that the woman was his mother. When I asked why his mother was there, Ken said that she was there to help him heal from her passing on during his teens.

I took him to his sacred place (see pages 156–157), asking his mother to be there as well. Ken spoke to his mother and complained that when she passed away he became the target of his father's abuse. Taking on the role of his mother, the response was: "Your father's abuse drove me to an early grave; but the most difficult part of passing on was leaving you. I'm sorry I couldn't be there any longer to protect you from your father, but my work in that life was done. You must bless me and release me, knowing that my love will always be with you even from the other side."

After going back and forth several times with the Gestalt role play dialogue, his mother praised him for not continuing the pattern of abuse with his children. Ken was able to finally say goodbye to his mother and release her.

The session was life changing, and the following month he enjoyed a successful regression therapy for the original concern.

### A Weighty Matter

Mary wanted to lose 50 pounds and keep it off. She told me that her weight had gone up and down like a yo-yo for over ten years, and that she'd lost several hundred pounds trying one diet after another.

The first two sessions helped her to stop eating as a coping technique for handling stress; but she still belonged to the "clean plate club" and was unable to stop eating desserts after dinner. Because it was not apparent whether to use regression or parts therapy, I employed ideomotor response questions. Her subconscious indicated "yes" for both imprint from an authority figure as well as a past event, so I chose to employ HRT to discover and release the causes. She also felt ashamed of herself for being overweight, so the affect bridge became the technique of choice.

My first surprise came after the affect bridge technique took her to a time in her early teens when two boys on the football team humiliated her in front of her friends, calling Mary a "fatty puss" (and worse names). This event hurt her deeply, making her embarrassed of her weight for the first time in her life. I wondered what this event had to do with an authority imprint; nonetheless, I asked guiding questions without assumptions in order to deal with what emerged. During the Gestalt, she vented considerable hate towards the two macho jerks who had ridiculed her, and then successfully released them by giving them their problem back. After confirming the release of that event, the subconscious indicated that more needed to be discovered and released. The source of her obsession with cleaning her plate required another regression session.

I used age regression at the second HRT session. Mary stopped me at age seven, telling me her mother was shouting at her for not eating all of her dinner. After she refused to finish her meal, her mother put her daughter's unfinished meal in the refrigerator, telling her she would have to eat the rest of her food the next day before she could have anything else. Meanwhile, Mary's mother served cheesecake to her father and brother, making Mary stay at the dinner table and watch. When she complained, her mother said, "You know the rules. Clean your plate, and you get dessert. Fail to finish a meal, and you are done for the day."

Now it became clear why she answered "yes" to authority imprint during the ideomotor response questions. The Gestalt with her mother lasted only a few moments, followed by subconscious confirmation of total release of the causes of overeating. Then I asked, "As a result of what was discovered and released, how will you best benefit in the here and now, or in the coming days, weeks and months?"

Mary's response during trance was that she ate dessert because her mother told her that it was a reward for cleaning the plate; so she would immediately resign from the clean plate club. I used suggestion and imagery to reinforce her ability to stop eating when full, releasing the excess food as she releases her excess pounds. In addition, I reminded her that after releasing the two football players and giving them their problem back, she could now feel good about who she is regardless of her weight; and that she was reducing because it was *her* decision, and not because of anyone else. In addition, I pulled out her list of personal benefits from a previous session and incorporated them into her imagery of success.

There are two ways to perceive Mary's childhood event at the dinner table: (1) the event was a combination of the initial sensitizing event and activating event for always cleaning her plate in order to get rewarded with dessert, and (2) failing to finish her dinner was the ISE and the AE happened minutes later when she watched others eat dessert while her mother imprinted Mary with the problem by scolding her.

The first regression to the event during her teens was a rare time when the subconscious takes a client to an SSE before going to either the ISE or AE of the presenting problem. However, that later event needed to be cleared because of the shame attached to her problem by the two football players. As an example of hypnosis being an art (subjective) more than a science (objective), we could also perceive Mary's humiliation for being overweight as the ISE for the shame that became attached to her problem.

Regardless of how we label the event from her early teens, an important lesson from this case history is that being overweight is often a multifaceted problem that may be linked with low self-esteem, guilt, shame and/or other issues. Often overweight clients need a series of sessions to deal with each issue attached to the problem, even though many clients might release some of those issues automatically when the core cause is discovered and released. Everyone is unique, and because being overweight is often a complex issue, numerous clients seeing me for weight loss over the years have required a series of sessions before enjoying lasting success.

# Epilogue

First, the authors would like to express appreciation to all hypnosis professionals and serious students of hypnotherapy who have chosen to read this book. Life is a series of learning experiences, and our objective has been to provide some important tools to help you learn additional effective ways of empowering your clients with hypnotic regression therapy.

We are all each other's teachers and students in life, and we can learn much from our clients as well as fellow professionals in the practice of professional hypnotherapy. We encourage you to keep that in mind when facilitating professional hypnosis, regardless of what techniques you employ. We have learned much from clients over the years, and we always endeavor to fine-tune our skills as a result of being aware of client successes as well as the "learning experiences" resulting from our mistakes.

This book is backed directly with over a half-century of combined experience from the two of us who wrote it; but indirectly it contains the wisdom and experience of several centuries of professional hypnotherapy when we consider the work of other professionals quoted and/ or referenced within these pages.

Yet in spite of all the above, there does not seem to be any perfect protocol for employing hypnotic regression therapy in a manner that will work for all clients all the time; otherwise someone most certainly would have discovered it by now. This is why we choose to consider HRT as an art rather than a science, and this is also why this book presents a variety of techniques.

If you are a hypnosis practitioner, we suggest that you use the techniques that fit both your style and the needs of your client—but always be willing to use another technique when one that you like does not bring the desired results. In other words, fit the technique to the client rather than vice versa. This is both wise and client centered, but it requires width and depth of training in the art of hypnotherapy. Also note that HRT is not a panacea for all problems, nor is it appropriate for every client requiring hypnotherapy. That is why we have included information on ideomotor response questioning as well as the seven psychodynamics of symptoms. The fact that some hypnosis professionals try to use HRT with all or most of their clients provides ammunition to the critics of regression therapy, lending some justifiable credibility to their complaints.

If you are a hypnotherapy instructor wishing to include hypnotic regression therapy in your training program, we trust that you will find this book to be a useful text. To enhance the learning experiences of your students, you may wish to facilitate role play exercises in your class. Pretend to be a client with a presenting problem requiring hypnotic regression therapy, and then ask your students to go through the various phases of HRT. If a student asks a leading question, makes an unwise choice and/or skips an important step, you can stop the role play and ask the class to suggest what could have been done for better results. I (Hunter) have found from experience that teaching regression in this manner helps students learn faster than simply having them watch demonstrations. While most students do not like being in the "hot seat" during these role play exercises, everyone learns—and I go around the room so that everyone has the opportunity to take the role of facilitator in the practice sessions.

If you are someone who has been skeptical of hypnotic regression therapy, we sincerely hope you have learned enough from this book to realize that client centered hypnotic regression has a place in hypnotherapy. Some HRT critics have gone so far as to claim that regression is like a dinosaur, outdated and obsolete. Our response to that claim is: If client centered regression still helps clients resolve problems, why should we even consider discarding it? While regression might result in problems if misapplied (such as inappropriate leading creating false memories, or sudden awakening during abreactions leaving the problem at the surface), we should not even consider throwing out the baby with the bathwater. Practitioners must have proper training so that they can appropriately integrate HRT into their case formulations and treatment plans, and so that they know how to manage abreactions and use them therapeutically.

Many clients over the years have experienced lasting success as a result of competent HRT, and our hope is that practitioners of hypnotic regression therapy will continue to improve their skills so that HRT continues to be used through the 21st century and beyond.

We agree that regression is not appropriate for all clients all the time, but client centered hypnotic regression therapy is the best technique available for some of the clients some of the time.

Upon request, and as time permits, we are available for workshops and/or mentoring.

Contact Bruce Eimer at: www.bruceeimer.com
Contact Roy Hunter at: www.royhunter.com

Or, if you prefer, you may go through Crown House Publishing.

# Appendix: Transcript of Regression Therapy Session

The regression transcript that follows took place with a hypnotherapist from California, who graciously gave permission for a transcript of her recorded session to be included in this book. Her name has been changed. Also, I would like to thank Scott Sandland (founder of hypnothoughts.com) for arranging the recording and allowing the use of the transcript in this book.

I (Roy Hunter) facilitated the session at a regression workshop in Southern California in June of 2011. Most of the pre-talk took place off camera. Prior to turning the camera on, we mutually decided to use age regression to discover the ISE. Although most of the intake happened off camera, the transcript starts during the preparation phase of regression, as described below ...

## Phase 1: Preparation

> **RH:** I know we talked off camera for a bit, but why don't you summarize for the viewers and the people in this room what you would like for me to help you with today?

> **DONNA:** I'd like for you to help me with perfection, and I have unrealistic expectations of myself and of others.

> **RH:** Is there anything else you feel I should know before we begin the process?

> **DONNA:** No.

> **RH:** OK ... very good. I'm going to set this down for a minute *[RH sets writing tablet down]* ... until I guide you deep enough for the regression. And of course *[moving into pre-talk ...]*, being in this class, you're aware that we don't always remember things exactly as they happen. Just like two children can witness a fight in the schoolyard, and then five minutes later give different versions to

a teacher. When emotions occur at the time of an event, the emotions can sometimes distort our perceptions; so when I guide you back in time in your mind, what you remember will be the way you perceive it. And your subconscious is responding to those perceptions as though they are real. My job is NOT to sort out fact from fantasy. Rather, it's to help you remember the perceptions, so that you can reframe those, and be released from whatever emotional attachments ...

*Client nods yes.*

**RH** (*continues pre-talk*): So if I ask you to either forgive or release somebody of an apology that you think they used to owe you, do you think you're going to be willing to do that?

**DONNA**: Yes.

**RH**: Good. Do you have any other questions before we start?

**DONNA**: No.

**RH**: What induction do you like? Whenever I do a session for a hypnosis professional, I give the hypnotherapist/client the choice of inductions.

**DONNA**: Progressive relaxation.

**RH**: OK, you got it ... and are you comfortable with your hand being touched?

**DONNA**: Yes.

*COMMENT: Remember to ask permission to touch BEFORE the induction; otherwise avoid any touch techniques throughout the entire session.*

**RH**: OK ... Now, are you going to be comfortable with your legs crossed?

**DONNA**: If I had some place to put them up with, that would be great, but ...

*Everyone in the room laughs ...*

COMMENT: *A number of hypnotherapists erroneously believe that a client cannot experience a successful session if he/she has either the arms or legs crossed. RH's experience has demonstrated otherwise. While crossing the arms or legs MIGHT become a source of discomfort, we can get around that potential obstacle by simply giving suggestions for the client to readjust to get more comfortable.*

**RH** (*induction begins*): You can feel free to readjust to get more comfortable anytime you wish; and whenever you are ready to begin, just close your eyes. Take a deep breath, and RELAX ... Imagine you're inhaling a sense of peace, and as you release the air from your lungs, you're releasing all the cares of the day, relaxing, and letting go ... and imagine you are seated comfortably in a beautiful peaceful place, with sights, sounds and sensations that are so calm, and so peaceful, that it gives you an increasing desire to just relax by imagining a relaxing sensation moving into your toes and feet.

(*Continues induction*): You can imagine feeling it, or seeing it, or experiencing it, in whatever way is comfortable to you. As you move this imaginary relaxation up through your ankles into your calves, every nerve and muscle responding to your desire to relax. The relaxation FLOWS up through your knees into your thighs ... gentle and soothing, comforting ... peaceful ... spreading, up through your hips, into your stomach muscles, circling your waist ... And you may notice how the mind can think many times faster than the spoken voice. So it's perfectly OK for your conscious mind to listen in, or drift and wander ... or do both ... while your subconscious is free to hear and respond to my voice.

(*Continuing induction*): As you go deeper with each breath you take, imagining more vividly a relaxation that feels more and more real ... spreading up through the small of your back, into the back of your shoulders and the top of your shoulders, just as though gentle fingers have given you a soothing back rub. And it just feels so relaxing it's easier and easier to go deeper and deeper relaxed ... Allowing the relaxation to flow down through your arms and elbows, right out your wrists, hands and fingers ... spreading through your neck and your scalp. Your forehead and temples relax.

Deeper and deeper, and your cheeks and jaw muscles relax ... every nerve and muscle relaxing completely, and it just feels so relaxing, it's easier to go deeper as I count from 10 to 1.

COMMENT: *Deepening starts at 4:40 in the video, beginning with counting down ...*

**RH**: Beginning with number 10 ... deeper with each number. Releasing all the cares of the day, relaxing into hypnotic peace, letting go. Number 9, deeper and deeper. Releasing, relaxing, letting go. Every sound you hear, especially the sound of my voice, making it easier and easier to go deeper and deeper until you reach your ideal depth. Number 8, deeper and deeper. Releasing, relaxing, letting go ... imagining a peaceful place, and you are becoming a part of the peace that you imagine. Number 7, deeper and deeper, relaxing physically. Deeper with each number, deeper with each breath. Number 6, deeper and deeper, relaxing mentally. Deeper because you choose, responding to my voice. Number 5, deeper and deeper, relaxing emotionally. The deeper you go, the better you feel, and the easier it is to go even deeper. Number 4, MUCH deeper ... just relaxing completely into the soothing tranquility of hypnotic peace. Even deeper on number 3, double the hypnosis or triple the trance ... releasing, relaxing, letting go. And on number 2, imagining more vividly ... sights, sounds, or sensations that are so calm, and so peaceful, and so tranquil, so serene, and so relaxing, it's easier and easier to go deeper and deeper on number 1 ... deeper yet. Even deeper ... waaaaaay down into the soothing tranquility of inner peace ... a very deep, inner peace.

COMMENT: *I give more suggestions for comfort since Donna still has her legs crossed ...*

**RH**: And any time you wish to readjust to get more comfortable, feel perfectly free to do so. Anytime throughout the entire session, if you wish to readjust to get more comfortable, feel free to do so. And as you allow yourself to go deeper listening to the sound of my voice, remember that in your imagination you can do anything that you wish. And it makes no difference whether your conscious mind is listening in or drifting and wandering, or doing both;

because your subconscious is free to hear and respond to my voice, and allow you to either enter the realm of hypnotic sleep, or you can let go into PROFOUND hypnosis.

*COMMENT: Eye catalepsy convincer given for additional deepening ...*

**RH**: In your imagination you can do anything you wish, so just imagine a sensation of drowsiness. You know what it feels like when you're sleepy. Imagine that sensation now, as though your eyelids are so heavy and droopy and drowsy, as though they're glued shut. So even if you try to open them you find they would rather stay shut. Stop trying, and either double the hypnosis or triple the trance. Going even deeper, releasing, relaxing, letting go.

*COMMENT: Elman floppy arm drop deepening technique employed ...*

**RH**: I'm going to pick up your left arm. Let me have the full weight of your arm. And when I release your arm, just release yourself into a deeper state *[releasing client's left arm]*, letting go. As I pick up your other arm and do the same thing, let me have the full weight of this arm, and when I release your arm you can release yourself into deep hypnosis, or you can let go into total trance ... releasing, relaxing, letting go *[releasing client's right arm]*, enjoying the journey as you go even deeper into the soothing tranquility of a very deep hypnotic peace. Every sound you hear, especially the sound of my voice, helping you go deeper and deeper. *[I retrieve the writing tablet.]*

*COMMENT: Ideomotor response signals established (just over nine minutes into session) ...*

**RH**: Donna, I'm going to ask your subconscious a series of questions; and if the answer is YES, please choose a finger or thumb that represents the YES response and indicate at this time. *[After response, I record it.]* Thank you. If I ask a question and the answer is N.O., please choose a different finger or thumb that represents the NO response. *[I record the NO response.]* Thank you. If I ask a question and the answer is either I'm not yet ready to disclose, or I don't know, please choose a different finger or thumb for that response. *[I record the IDK response.]* Thank you.

*COMMENT: One Hundred to One scale started ... Note that even though the client told me off camera that she already had a peaceful place, it would have been wise for me to confirm it before moving on.*

**RH**: Now on a scale of the number 100 down to the number 1, 100 representing awake with your eyes closed, and number 1 is ABSOLUTELY as deep as you can go in hypnosis without falling asleep. 50 is half way, medium. If you are 50 or deeper, please move the YES finger. *[YES finger moves.]* Very good. Are you 40 or deeper? *[YES finger moves.]* Excellent. Are you 30 or deeper? *[YES finger moves.]*

*COMMENT: Regardless of the response to "30 or deeper," we can continue with the next question.*

**RH**: Are you deep enough to continue the next phase of the session? *[YES finger moves.]* Excellent.

*COMMENT: To reduce the risk of an analytical client from resisting the regression and/or emerging from hypnosis, I usually add the following suggestion ...*

**RH**: Any time I touch the back of your hand and say "deep hypnosis" allow yourself to return to this level of hypnosis *[touching back of client's hand while giving suggestion]*. And if this suggestion is acceptable at all levels of consciousness, please move the YES finger.

*YES finger moves.*

**RH**: Thank you. Allow yourself to remain in deep hypnosis, or at your ideal level of trance throughout the remainder of this journey.

## Phase 2: Regression Techniques to Discover the Cause

**RH** (*defining problem previously stated by client*): And as we move into the next phase of the session, I'm going to ask your subconscious a question regarding the problem you stated before this journey began ... that problem of wanting to be perfect, of making demands on yourself and others.

**RH**: (*using age regression*): Did the origin of this problem happen at age 30 or earlier? *[YES finger moves.]* At age 25 or earlier? *[YES finger moves.]* At or before age 20? *[YES finger moves.]*

*COMMENT: While I normally start counting backwards at either 25 or 20, this time I chose to start at age 15 in order to save time on camera … but it is optional to start individual numbers as high as age 30. Also remember that it is acceptable to start age regression at Zero and count forwards.*

**RH**: At or before age 15? *[YES finger moves.]* As I count backwards, please stop me or move the YES finger when I get to a very significant age … when I get to the age of very high importance, either stop me or move the YES finger. 14 … 13 … 12, getting smaller, younger … 11 … Age 10 … 9 … 8 … 7 … stop me when I get to a very important age … 6 … 5 … 4 …

*Client's IDK finger moves at the Number four …*

**RH**: At age 4, something important happened … be there. What do you see, hear, or feel? *[No response …]* Where are you? … and what's happening? *[Still no response …]* Allow your subconscious to take you where you need to go … it's safe to speak …

*Client finally responds after a long pause …*

**RH**: What do you see, hear, or feel?

*Client speaks too softly to understand …*

**RH**: Pardon?

**DONNA**: Garage.

**RH**: Garage? What's happening in the garage?

*Client mumbles something about cousins there …*

**RH**: Your cousins are there?

**DONNA**: One.

**RH**: One cousin?

**DONNA**: Uh-huh.

**RH**: And what is your cousin doing?

**DONNA**: He's taking his penis out.

**RH**: What happens now?

**DONNA**: He wants me to take my panties off.

**RH**: And what do you do?

**DONNA**: I do what he tells me.

## Phase 3: Abreactions and Release

COMMENT: *When we reach the point where abreactions are either apparent or suppressed, we cross the bridge from Phase 2 into Phase 3.*

**RH**: And what happens now?

**DONNA**: He's talking to me.

COMMENT: *Client suppresses her abreactions, so I ask the following question in order to invite abreactions ...*

**RH**: How does this make you feel?

**DONNA**: I want to be his friend ... *[Facial expression indicates presence of emotions during pause ...]*

**RH**: What happens next?

**DONNA**: I don't know; we're just there ... *[long pause ...]*

**RH**: Move forward in time to when something important happens ... what's happening now?

*Client mumbles ...*

**RH**: Pardon?

**DONNA**: We build our house.

**RH**: You build a house?

**DONNA**: Yea, my parents are building a house.

COMMENT: *Since there are no further abreactions, client is taken to peaceful place to prepare for informed child technique and Gestalt role play in order to release the event ...*

**RH**: All right, go to your peaceful place ... be in your peaceful place for a moment. *[Informed child technique ...]* And with all of your present adult wisdom, knowledge, understanding, experience, be the four-year-old, but with your present adult mind. And now go back to that garage with your cousin, with your adult mind helping your four-year-old child. What is your new perception and new understanding of this event?

**DONNA**: I could've said NO. I could've left.

**RH** (*employing Gestalt role play ...*): Imagine your cousin is in front of you right now, and you can tell him anything you like. He has to listen to you. He must listen until you are finished speaking. Tell him how you feel about what he did ... how it affected you then, and in the years that followed. "It made me feel like ..."

**DONNA**: You made me feel like I had to do whatever you said to make me like you.

**RH**: What else do you want to say to him?

**DONNA**: I'm just a girl ... *[abreactions become more apparent ...]* I was only a little girl. 'Cause of that, you screwed up my life *[abreactions become moderate]* ...

**RH**: Feel free to use the tissue as desired ... *[client uses tissue handed to her by a classmate ...]* Is there anything else you want to say to him before he responds?

*Client shakes head "No."*

**RH**: Now, be your cousin. Donna said that you screwed up her life. What do you say to Donna?

**DONNA** (*speaking as cousin*): I'm sorry. I'm a stupid kid. I didn't think about my behavior. I didn't care. No one cared about me, so I didn't care about anyone else.

**RH**: Be Donna again. Your cousin said he's sorry. He said he didn't care because nobody cared about him. Do you understand him now?

**DONNA**: Yea.

COMMENT: *Some people equate "forgive" with "condone," so note the wording as I seek release …*

**RH** (*seeking release*): Without condoning what he did, do you forgive him or release him from the apology he used to owe you?

**DONNA**: Yes.

**RH**: And do you forgive yourself for carrying that hurt around all these years?

*Client nods her head, whispering "Yes."*

**RH**: Very good. Go to your peaceful place.

COMMENT: *Once a client releases a person, it is time to guide him/her back to the peaceful place in order to confirm release.*

**RH** (confirming release of that event): I would like to ask your subconscious to respond with the appropriate finger response. Has that event and your cousin been successfully released?

*YES finger moves.*

COMMENT: *If the NO or IDK finger had moved, I would have asked Donna if she needed to speak to anyone else regarding the event. Sometimes a client wishes to role play with a parent or someone else even if said person was not present during the event. When two or more people are involved in the event, the client often needs to experience Gestalt with more than one person.*

**RH**: Is there anything else that must be discovered and released?

*YES finger moves.*

**RH**: And are you ready to do so at this time?

*YES finger moves again.*

*COMMENT: In a private session, watch the time. More often than not, a second regression must be scheduled at a subsequent session simply for time's sake. (Less than 20 minutes have passed in Donna's regression session.) However, when time does permit a second regression, I ask the client's permission before continuing, as the client often needs to process the first regression before moving on.*

**RH** (*attempting another regression*): Then from that garage, move either forward or backward in time to a very significant event; moving either forward or backward in time to a very significant event involving the desire to be perfect ... a very important event. 3, 2, 1, BE there. What's happening? Where are you?

*Long pause ... no response; changing regression techniques to affect bridge since emotions occurred during first regression ...*

**RH**: Can you go into the feeling of what it's like when you want to be perfect, when you want to do good? Go into those feelings. You know how you feel when you want perfection out of yourself or out of somebody else. And as I count from 1 to 10, go into those feelings. 1, going into those feelings more on 2. 3, allow yourself to feel those feelings as much as you safely can. 4, 5. You know what it feels like when you demand perfection from yourself or somebody else. 6, taking the feeling, go into those feelings as much as you safely can when I get to 10.

*COMMENT: Client starts abreacting, so I accelerate the count ...*

**RH**: 7 8, 9, 10. As I count backwards go back to the first time you felt those feelings, 10, 9, 8, WAY back. 7, 6, 5, 4, to where your subconscious needs you to go. 3, 2, 1, BE there. What's happening, where are you?

**DONNA** (*moves YES finger and speaks ...*): It's so critical.

**RH**: What's critical?

**DONNA** (*mumbles, then continues ...*): They think they were right.

**RH**: Where are you right now?

**DONNA**: Grandparents' house.

**RH**: Your grandparents?

**DONNA** (*abreacts and continues …*): I can't do anything right. They say they work so hard.

**RH**: How old are you right now?

**DONNA**: Nine.

**RH**: And where are you?

**DONNA**: In the house.

**RH**: Which house?

**DONNA**: The new house.

**RH** (*verifying …*): The new house?

*COMMENT: If you are not totally certain what the client said, it is acceptable to repeat what you believe the client said in order to verify what you thought you heard …*

**DONNA**: They're being mean.

**RH**: Pardon?

*COMMENT: Often a client speaks very softly. If you cannot under-stand what he/she says, it is OK to either ask the client to repeat the answer or say "Pardon?"*

**DONNA**: They're being mean.

**RH** (*verifying*): They're being mean?

**DONNA**: Uh huh …

**RH**: How are they being mean?

**DONNA**: They're saying mean things.

**RH**: Do you know why they're saying mean things to you?

**DONNA**: 'Cause they can't control me.

**RH** (*verifying …*): They can't control you?

**DONNA**: And they don't like that.

**RH**: How are they trying to control you?

**DONNA**: They want me to do what they want me to do, and I won't do it. They say I'm outspoken, and I misbehave, and no one's going to love me, and my parents didn't love me, so ...

**RH**: And how does this make you feel?

**DONNA**: It hurts!

**RH**: Go to your peaceful place. And just like before, allow your highest and best wisdom, knowledge, understanding, training and experience to assist the 9-year-old. In a moment I'm going to ask you to go back to the house as a 9-year-old, but with all of your present adult wisdom, knowledge, understanding, training and experience. With the adult mind, be the 9-year-old. What's your new perception of the way you're being treated?

**DONNA**: They just don't understand me. They're not bright; they're not very smart.

**RH**: Imagine they're sitting in front of you now; but this time they have to listen to everything you want to say. Which one do you want to talk to first?

**DONNA**: I want to talk to both of them at the same time.

**RH** (*verifying ...*): At the same time? OK.

**DONNA** (*speaking to grandparents ...*): I thought you were sup-posed to protect me. I thought I was able to come to you and tell you when things were wrong. I thought you wanted me ... but you didn't. You wanted perfection. You wanted me to be something I couldn't be. You weren't willing to accept me for who I was. And you didn't have to tell me that my parents didn't love me. You don't know that. You just wanted me to stay there with you while you were so mean to me. And you didn't protect me when I needed your protection. You put me in bad situations. And I tried so hard to be what you wanted. I could never live up to ... 'cause you didn't know what you wanted. And I tried so hard.

**RH**: Is there anything else you want to say to them before they respond?

**DONNA**: No.

**RH**: Which one do you want to respond? Who do you want to speak in response to you?

**DONNA**: My grandmother.

**RH**: All right. Be your grandmother. Your granddaughter says that she was unwanted, and that you tried to make her a perfectionist. She said some other things about how hurtful you were. How do you respond to her?

**DONNA** (*as grandmother speaking to Donna ...*): I'm sorry. I didn't know that I was hurting you. I just was old, and I had your responsibility. And I didn't want you to leave me and look for your mother and your dad. I wanted you to stay with me. I loved you, and I still do; and I'm sorry. I didn't have good parenting skills. I treated you the same way I was treated. And I'm sorry I didn't protect you. I didn't know what else to do. And I'm sorry all those bad things happened to you.

**RH**: Now be Donna. Your grandmother is sorry. Are you willing to forgive her or release her from the apology she used to owe you?

**DONNA**: Yes.

**RH**: And do you forgive yourself for carrying the hurt all these years?

**DONNA**: Yea.

**RH**: Very good. Do you also wish to speak to your grandfather?

**DONNA**: Yes ... bad man, a very bad man. He shouldn't have been allowed to walk the face of the earth. He did some very bad things ... mean, bad. Me, and all the other women in our family. [*Now speaking to grandfather ...*] You hit my grandmother. She couldn't leave you. She hears so bad. You're a very mean man.

**RH**: What else do you want to say to him?

**DONNA**: Because of you, I lived in this life, just trying to get love … trying to find love in all the wrong places. Because of you, my sister left me all alone … and I thought it was my fault. She was only trying to escape you.

**RH**: Anything else you wish to say before he responds?

**DONNA**: Nope.

**RH**: All right, be the grandfather. Your granddaughter just said that you did some mean things, and you hurt her. How do you respond to your granddaughter?

**DONNA** (*speaking as grandfather to Donna …*): I'm sorry. I don't know how to love; I never did. I never learned. I was a bad parent, and I shouldn't have done the things I did to you and your sister.

**RH**: Be Donna. Your grandfather said he's sorry, and he didn't know how to love. Is there anything you wish to say to him before you forgive him or release him?

**DONNA**: No.

**RH**: Are you willing to forgive or release him without condoning, or release him from the apology he used to owe you?

**DONNA**: Yes.

**RH**: And do you forgive yourself for carrying the anger and the hurt all these years?

**DONNA**: Yes.

**RH**: (*returning client to peaceful place to confirm release …*): Very good. Go back to your peaceful place. *[Pause …]* Have you now successfully released that event, as well as your grandparents? Please answer with the appropriate finger response.

*YES finger moves …*

**RH**: Very good. Is there anything else that must be discovered and released?

*Both YES and NO fingers move …*

**RH**: Both fingers moved. Would you please answer again: has that problem and its causes been successfully released?

*YES finger moves …*

**RH**: Very good.

COMMENT: *Once we confirm release of both the problem and its causes, we can now move into Phase 4, Subconscious Relearning (or reprogramming), using suggestion and imagery, and/or metaphors, NLP, EFT, or other techniques to help reprogram the subconscious.*

## Phase 4: Subconscious Relearning

**RH**: As a result of what was discovered and released, how will you best benefit in the here and now, and the coming days, weeks and months?

**DONNA**: I know I was loved, and they just didn't know how to show it.

**RH**: Very good. *[Asking appropriate leading question regarding relearning …]* Will that also empower you to love yourself more?

**DONNA**: Yes.

COMMENT: *Inappropriate leading questions are those which create false perceptions as to the cause(s) of a client's problem. However, once the subconscious cause(s) are discovered and released, it is OK to ask leading questions regarding the RESOLUTION of the client's problem.*

**RH**: Very good. Are you willing to let it be OK to be the best that you can be instead of trying to be perfect?

**DONNA**: Yes.

**RH**: It's so much easier to be the best that you can be instead of trying to be perfect … because by simply being the best you can be, one day your best is better than another day, and it's OK. And it's OK to love yourself. That's the other half of the golden rule, so allow it to be OK to love yourself enough to be your own best friend. And if this is acceptable at all levels of consciousness, move the YES finger.

*YES finger moves ...*

**RH**: Very good. As a result of this, how will you best be empowered in the coming days, weeks and months?

**DONNA**: I'll be tolerant of myself. I'll love myself. I won't put unrealistic expectations on myself.

**RH**: Very good. And will this make it easy for you not to put unrealistic expectations on others, so that you can be tolerant of others as well?

**DONNA**: Yes.

**RH**: (*giving suggestions to enhance subconscious relearning ...*): Very good. Allow yourself to be the best you can be so that it's easier and easier every day to enjoy your own ideal empowerment. And every time you find yourself making a good decision, it's easier to make another good decision; because like a muscle that's used is stronger with use, your power of choice is stronger with use. So as you make wise choices about yourself and others, it's easier to make more wise choices. And if you wish to establish a trigger to connect to your best wisdom, knowledge, understanding, training and experience in any given situation, you can touch your thumb to a finger that you choose as your TOLERANT trigger.

*Client touches thumb to index finger ...*

**RH**: Very good. It allows you to connect to your best wisdom, knowledge, understanding, training and experience ... to be tolerant, but also to make a wise choice that's the best choice for everybody concerned ... but you include yourself in what's best for everybody concerned. And you have the power to make it so, and so it is. And if there are any other additional suggestions for self-empowerment that a part of your subconscious or inner mind wishes to give you, just speak them out loud as affirmations.

**DONNA**: Peace, and joy.

**RH** (*verifying ...*): Peace and joy ... excellent. You can allow either or both of those words to be automatic reminders for you to be the best that you can be ... to find the peace and the joy in your life, and to have the power to make it so. And so it is.

## Phase 5: Concluding the Session

**RH**: In a moment I'm going to count back from 1 to 5; but before I do, just enjoy being in your peaceful place ... allowing all of the suggestions that benefit and empower you, and only those suggestions that benefit and empower you to merge into your mind, becoming a part of you because you choose. And when you again hear the sound of my voice, it will be almost time to come back.

*Client has 30 seconds of silence ...*

In a moment you can start returning gradually and gently to conscious awareness; and it doesn't matter whether the moments of silence seemed like a few seconds or five minutes or more. What's important is that you now have the freedom to be the best you that you can be. Number 1 ... slowly, gently, gradually returning to conscious awareness; becoming aware of the room and the here and now, and the chair that you're sitting on, and the friends in this room with you. Number 2 ... imagine feeling the way you wish to feel for the rest of the day and evening. Feeling good about yourself ... finding it's easier every day in every way to find the peace and the joy in your life. Knowing that you have the power to make it so, because it's so much easier to be your best. And on 3 give yourself the idea that any time and every time you get behind the wheel of a motor vehicle, you are alert and responsive to any and all traffic and road situations. Stretching a little bit on number 4. And eyes open on 5 when you are ready.

*Client stretches and opens her eyes.*

**RH**: (*starting debrief ...*): Amazing stuff, isn't it?

*Long pause, with no response from client as she wipes her eyes and face with fresh tissues ...*

**RH**: How do you feel?

**DONNA**: Oh, like I've been crying.

**RH**: Yes, indeed. Do you feel more empowered now?

**DONNA**: Uh huh.

**RH**: (*to class*): Notice the appropriate leading question?

**DONNA**: Yes. I feel like I have some answers ... that I didn't have before.

**RH**: Indeed, you do have answers you didn't have before. More important, in addition to the answers, you also have the appropriate release which your subconscious confirmed ... and along with that, the empowerment to be your best. Congratulations on a great breakthrough!

Thank you.

*AFTER BREAK ...*

Donna told the class that what emerged was a total surprise. She never thought about the ISE having an impact on her problem. She knew it happened, but said she never discussed it with anyone, neither in previous sessions nor in counseling. Later that evening, she told several of us at dinner that the session was quite helpful.

# References

American Psychiatric Association. 1994. *Diagnostic and Statistical Manual of Mental Disorders, Fourth Edition* (DSM-IV). Arlington, VA: APA.

Banyan, C. D. 2005. The Banyan Glossary of Hypnosis Terms. Available at www.hypnosiscenter.com/hypnosis-definitions.htm (accessed November 2, 2011).

Banyan, C. D. 2009. Ten Keys for Successful Age Regression Work. Available at www.calbanyan.com/archives/2009/03/13/hypnosis-training-video-podcast-108-ten-keys-for-success ful-age-regression-work (accessed August 19, 2011).

Banyan, C. D. and Kein, G. F. 2001. *Hypnosis and Hypnotherapy: Basic to Advanced Techniques for the Professional.* Tustin, CA: Abbot Publishing House.

Barber, J. 1996. *Hypnosis and Suggestion in the Treatment of Pain: A Clinical Guide.* New York: W. W. Norton.

Barber, J. and Adrian, C. 1982. *Psychological Approach to the Management of Pain.* New York: Brunner/Mazel.

Beck, A. T. 1979. *Cognitive Therapy and the Emotional Disorders.* New York: Penguin.

Bowman, C. 1998. *Children's Past Lives.* New York: Bantam Books.

Boyne, G. 1989. *Transforming Therapy: A New Approach to Hypnotherapy.* Glendale, CA: Westwood Publishing.

Bradshaw, J. 1988. *Bradshaw on the Family: A Revolutionary Way of Self-Discovery.* Deerfield Beach, FL: Health Communications.

Brown, D., Hammond, D. C. and Scheflin, A. W. 1998. *Memory, Trauma Treatment, and the Law.* New York: W. W. Norton.

Callahan, R. & Trubo, R. 2002. *Tapping the healer within: Using Thought-Field Therapy to instantly conquer your fears, anxieties and emotional distress*. New York: McGraw-Hill.

Cheek, D. 1993. *Hypnosis: The Application of Ideomotor Techniques*. Boston, MA: Allyn & Bacon.

Cheek, D. B. and LeCron, L. M. 1968. *Clinical Hypnotherapy*. New York: Grune & Stratton.

Churchill, R. 2002. *Regression Hypnotherapy: Transcripts of Transformation*. Santa Rosa, CA: Transforming Press.

Churchill, R. 2008. *Catharsis in Regression Hypnotherapy*, Vol. II: *Transcripts of Transformation*. Santa Rosa, CA: Transforming Press.

Colgrove, M., Bloomfield, H. H. and McWilliams, P. 1993. *How to Survive the Loss of a Love*. Los Angeles, CA: Mary Book/Prelude Press.

Durbin, P. G. 2001. Beware of False Memories: Revised. Available at www.durbinhypnosis.com/falsememdurbin.htm (accessed August 2, 2011).

Eastburn, D. 2007. *The Power of the Past: Transformational Replay: State-of-the-Art Hypnotic Regression Therapy*. Victoria, BC: Trafford Publishing.

Eimer, B. N. 2007. *Hypnotize Yourself Out of Pain Now!* Oakland, CA: New Harbinger Publications.

Eimer, B. N. and Freeman, A. 1996. *Pain Management Psychotherapy: A Practical Guide*. New York: John Wiley.

Eimer, B. N. and Gravitz, M. A. 2007. Clinical and Forensic Hypnosis. In F. Dattilio and R. Sadoff (eds.), *Mental Health Experts: Roles and Qualifications for Court*, 2nd edn. Mechanicsburg, PA: Pennsylvania Bar Institute, pp. 157–173.

Ellis, A. and Harper, R. A. 1975. *A New Guide to Rational Living*. Chatsworth, CA: Wilshire Book Co.

Elman, D. 1984. *Hypnotherapy*. Glendale, CA: Westwood Publishing.

Emmerson, G. 2003. *Ego State Therapy*. Carmarthen, Wales: Crown House Publishing.

Erickson, M. H., Hershman, S. and Secter, I. I. 1961. *The Practical Application of Medical and Dental Hypnosis*. New York: Julian Press.

Ewin, D. M. 2009. *101 Things I Wish I'd Known When I Started Using Hypnosis*. Carmarthen, Wales: Crown House Publishing.

Ewin, D. M. and Eimer, B. N. 2006. *Ideomotor Signals for Rapid Hypnoanalysis: A How-To Manual*. Springfield, IL: Charles C. Thomas.

Fiore, E. 1995. *The Unquiet Dead: A Psychologist Treats Spirit Possession*. New York: Ballantine Books.

Hall, J. 1976. *Classical Conditioning and Instrumental Learning: A Contemporary Approach*. Philadelphia, PA: Lippincott.

Hammond, D. C., Garver, R. B., Mutter, C. B., Crasilneck, H. B., Frischolz, E., Gravitz, M. A. Hibler, N. S., Olson, J., Scheflin, A., Spiegel, D. and Wester, W. 1995. *Clinical Hypnosis and Memory: Guidelines for Clinicians and for Forensic Hypnosis*. Des Plaines, IL: American Society of Clinical Hypnosis.

Howell, M. 2011. Forensic Application of Hypnosis. Available at www.marxhowell.com/Forensic-Application-of-Hypnosis-Howell.html (accessed August 23, 2011).

Hunter, C. R. 1995/2000/2007. *The Art of Hypnotherapy: Part II of Diversified Client-Centered Hypnosis, Based on the Teachings of Charles Tebbetts* (edn. 1, 2, 3). Dubuque, IA: Kendall/Hunt Publishing Company.

Hunter, C. R. 2005. *Hypnosis for Inner Conflict Resolution: Introducing Parts Therapy*. Carmarthen, Wales: Crown House Publishing.

Hunter, C. R. 2010a. *The Art of Hypnosis*, 3rd edn. Carmarthen, Wales: Crown House Publishing.

Hunter, C. R. 2010b. *The Art of Hypnotherapy*, 4th edn. Carmarthen, Wales: Crown House Publishing.

James, T. and Woodsmall, W. 1988. *Time Line Therapy and the Basis of Personality*. Capitola, CA: Meta Publications.

Jelenik, P. 2008. Number of Troops Suffering from PTSD up 50%. *Marine Corps Times*, May 27, 2008. Available at www.marinecorpstimes.com/news/2008/05/ap_ptsd_052708 (accessed November 1, 2011).

Kinchin, D. 2011. What is Post Traumatic Stress Disorder? Available at www.burnsurvivorsttw.org/articles/ptsd1.html (accessed November 1, 2011).

Kubler-Ross, E. and Kessler, D. 2007. *On Grief and Grieving: Finding the Meaning of Grief Through the Five Stages of Loss*. New York: Scribner.

Lazarus, A. A. 1989. *The Practice of Multimodal Therapy: Systematic, Comprehensive, and Effective Psychotherapy*. Baltimore, MD: Johns Hopkins University Press.

LeCron, L. M. 1964. *Self-Hypnotism: The Technique and Its Use in Daily Living*. Upper Saddle River, NJ: Prentice-Hall.

Loftus, E. and Ketcham, K. 1996. *The Myth of Repressed Memory: False Memories*. New York: St. Martin's Griffin.

Prophet, E. C. and Prophet, E. L. 1997. *Reincarnation: The Missing Link in Christianity*. Gardiner, MT: Summit University Press.

Quigley, D. 2011. *The Alchemy of Healing: Healing Your Body and Your Life with Hypnosis Therapy*. Santa Rosa, CA: Alchemy Institute of Hypnosis.

Quimby, P. P. 1961. *The Quimby Manuscripts*, ed. H. W. Dresser. Secaucus, NJ: Citadel Press.

Quimby, P. P. 1988. *Phineas Parkhurst Quimby: The Complete Writings*, 3 vols, ed. Ervin Seale. Marina del Rey, CA: DeVorss & Co.

Rossi, E. L. 1993. *The Psychobiology of Mind–Body Healing: New Concepts of Therapeutic Hypnosis*, rev. edn. New York: W. W. Norton.

Rossi, E. L. and Cheek, D. B. 1994. *Mind–Body Therapy: Methods of Ideodynamic Healing in Hypnosis*. New York: W. W. Norton.

Rothman, S. 2011. Trance after Hypnotherapy. Available at http://rothmanhypnosis.wordpress.com/2011/09/25/trance-after-hypnotherapy (accessed September 27, 2011).

Scheflin, A.W. (2012). How not to conduct a forensic hypnosis interview. *American Journal of Clinical Hypnosis*, 54 (4).

Scheflin, A. W. and Shapiro, J. L. 1989. *Trance on Trial*. New York: Guilford Press.

Schimelpfening, N. 2008. Almost 1 in 5 Troops Suffer from Depression, PTSD. Available at http://depression.about.com/b/2008/04/22/almost-1-in-5-troops-suffer-from-depression-ptsd.htm (accessed November 1, 2011).

Shapiro, F. 2011. Eye Movement Desensitization and Reprocessing. Available at www.emdr.com (accessed November 1, 2011).

Smith, M. and Segal, J. 2011. Post-Traumatic Stress Disorder (PTSD): Symptoms, Treatment, and Self-Help. Available at http://helpguide.org/mental/post_traumatic_stress_disorder_symptoms_treatment.htm (accessed October 17, 2011).

Spiegel, H. and Spiegel, D. 2004. *Trance and Treatment: Clinical Uses of Hypnosis*, 2nd edn. Arlington, VA: American Psychiatric Publishing.

Stevenson, Ian. 1987. *Children who Remember Previous Lives*. Charlottesville, VA: University Press of Virginia.

Tebbetts, C. 1985. *Miracles on Demand*. Dexter, MI: Thompson Shore (out of print).

Tilles, Y. 2011. Judaism and Reincarnation. Available at http://southerncrossreview.org/68/judaism-reincarnation2.htm (accessed February 10, 2012).

United States, Department of Veterans Affairs. 2007. Treatment of PTSD. Available at www.ptsd.va.gov/public/pages/treatment-ptsd.asp (accessed October 17, 2011).

Watkins, J. G. 1949. *Hypnotherapy of War Neuroses: A Clinical Psychologist's Casebook*. New York: Ronald Press.

Watkins, J. G. 1978. *The Therapeutic Self: Developing Resonance—Key to Effective Relationships*. New York, NY: Human Sciences Press.

Watkins, J. G. and Watkins, H. H. 1997. *Ego States: Theory and Therapy*. New York: W.W. Norton.

Weiss, B. L. 1988. *Many Lives, Many Masters: The True Story of a Prominent Psychiatrist, His Young Patient, and the Past-Life Therapy That Changed Both Their Lives*. New York: Simon & Schuster.

Weiss, B. L. 1993. *Through Time into Healing*. New York: Simon & Schuster.

Weiss, B. 1996. *Only Love Is Real: A Story of Soulmates Reunited*. New York: Warner Books.

Wester, W. C. and Hammond, D. C. (2011). Solving Crimes with Hypnosis. *American Journal of Clinical Hypnosis* 53(4), 249–263.

Winkler, A. 1976. *Reincarnation and the Interim between Lives*. Springfield, LA: St. John's University Publications.

Wolpe, J. 1973. *Practice of Behavior Therapy*, 2nd edn. New York: Permagon Press.

Woolger, R. J. 1988. *Other Lives, Other Selves: A Jungian Psychotherapist Discovers Past Lives*. New York: Bantam Books.

Worden, J. W. 2009. *Grief Counseling and Grief Therapy: A Handbook for the Mental Health Practitioner*, 4th edn. New York: Springer Publishing.

Yapko, M. D. 1995. *Essentials of Hypnosis*. New York: Brunner/Mazel.

Zanuso, B. 1986. *The Young Freud: The Origins of Psychoanalysis in Late Nineteenth-Century Viennese Culture*. Oxford, NY: Blackwell Publishers.

Zarren, J. I. and Eimer, B. N. 2002. *Brief Cognitive Hypnosis: Facilitating the Change of Dysfunctional Behavior*. New York: Springer Publishing.

# Index

abreactions 1–2, 7, 29, 37, 93–94, 101, 105, 107–111, 127, 134, 140, 147–149, 158–159, 188–189, 198–199
  intense 86, 108–110, 118, 121, 147, 158–159, 166, 179
  minimal 108, 110
  moderate 108–109, 199
  past life 129–139
  suppressed 110, 198
  *see also* release
activating event (AE) 27
affect bridge 27, 58, 79, 85–91, 103, 105, 118, 133, 169, 178–182, 184, 201
anxiety 9, 50, 134–135, 163–168, 171
art, of hypnosis 7, 14, 17, 60

Bandler, Richard 8
Banyan, Cal 5, 51, 88, 90
Barber, Joseph 64
bereavement, *see* grief
body lights imagery 172
Boyne, Gil 4–5, 107, 112
Bradshaw, John 127
bridge across the river of time 143

cause(s) 2–3, 5–7, 18, 20–24, 26, 28, 37, 40, 44–45, 49–50, 54, 79–80, 82–84, 86, 97, 100–101, 105, 107, 110, 114, 119, 121–124, 126–127, 134, 136, 146, 153, 160, 168–169, 176, 178, 180–182, 186, 196, 199, 206
Cheek, David 4–5, 11, 15, 171–172
chronic pain 169, 171
Churchill, Randal 5, 21, 107, 112
claustrophobia 103, 114
cloud technique 140
cognitive-behavioral therapy (CBT) x, xix, 9–11, 23, 166–167

control panel of light switches 174
cornerstones of hypnotherapy, *see* objectives of hypnotherapy
crystal hall technique 141

debrief 125, 208
deck of time 101
dissociation 107–109, 165
Durbin, Paul 44

ego state therapy 20–21, 26, 34, 119
ego strengthening 125
elevator through time 103, 142
empathy, importance of 12–13, 45
Elman, Dave 5, 78
Emmerson, Gordon 21, 34, 49
Erickson, Milton 11, 15
Ewin, Dabney vii, 4, 12, 26, 54
eye movement desensitization and reprocessing (EMDR) 10

false memory syndrome; *see also* past life regression 1–3, 7, 21, 33, 36–37, 43–45, 47–49, 57, 81, 131, 136, 146, 188
fear
  of birds 29
  of flying 2, 26, 28, 89, 126, 134–135, 181
  of snakes 118
  of water 133, 177–178
forensic hypnosis 3, 34, 43–45, 48, 99–101
forgiveness 22, 114, 148–149
Freud, Sigmund 10

Gestalt role play 112–113, 116–117, 121, 148, 154–155, 157, 159–161, 178, 180, 183, 199–200
grief 153–154, 158–161